TEAS® TEST OF ESSENTIAL ACADEMIC SKILLS

CRASH COURSE®

Research & Education Association

Visit our website at: www.rea.com

Research & Education Association
61 Ethel Road West
Piscataway, New Jersey 08854
E-mail: info@rea.com

TEAS® CRASH COURSE®

TABLE of CONTENTS

ABOUT THIS BOOK

REA's *TEAS Crash Course* is the first book of its kind for the time-crunched studier or any nursing school applicant who wants a quick refresher before taking the Test of Essential Academic Skills, or TEAS. This *Crash Course* is based upon a careful analysis of the exam's content and actual test questions.

The *TEAS Crash Course* provides a review specifically targeted to what you really need to know to ace the exam. In Chapter 1, the author describes the format and the content of the TEAS, shares proven test-taking strategies, and lets you determine how well-suited you are to the nursing profession.

Chapter 2 covers Reading Comprehension, a topic that comprises more than 25% of the 150 total questions on the TEAS test. Chapter 3 reviews Language topics, such as Grammar, Spelling, Punctuation, and Vocabulary; while chapters 4 and 5 give you a review of Basic Math concepts: Measurement, and Algebra. The final two chapters are devoted to the largest part of the TEAS: nearly 1/3 of all the questions you will answer on the final exam focus on the topics of Life Science (Chapter 6) and Physical Science (Chapter 7).

Note that all of the chapters give you a targeted content review in an outline format, along with sample problems that test what you've just reviewed. This format will help you build your confidence and your understanding of the topics as you study.

No matter how or when you prepare for the TEAS, REA's *Crash Course* will empower you to study efficiently and strategically, so you can get a high score.

Good luck on the TEAS!

To check your test readiness for the TEAS, either before or after studying this *Crash Course*, take our **FREE online practice exam**. To access your free exam, visit *www.rea.com/studycenter* and enter your exclusive access code found in the front inside cover of this book. This true-to-format test features automatic scoring, detailed answer explanations, and diagnostic feedback to help you identify your strengths and weaknesses and get you ready for test day.

A NOTE FROM OUR AUTHOR

The basic approach of this *TEAS Crash Course* is simple: the targeted content review covers exactly what you need to know for the TEAS. You won't waste valuable study time slogging through long paragraphs, complicated explanations, and endless lists of items to memorize. The sample problems in the book will demonstrate how you should answer the types of questions you can expect to see on the TEAS.

Before you start studying, ask yourself: how prepared are you to take the TEAS? Some students will be ready to take the test the minute they pick up this book, while another segment of test-takers may be completely underprepared. Most test-takers will fall somewhere between these two extremes. Maybe you're more confident (and competent) in some areas than you are in others. So what should you do? There are four ways to study with this *Crash Course*. Pick the one that works best for you.

1. The Systematic Approach – Start at the beginning and go through the entire book, chapter by chapter, problem by problem, not skipping anything, and making sure you cover every topic thoroughly.

2. The Strength Approach – Review the sections that you feel are your strong points, then work into areas that give you trouble. Starting with your strengths will give you the confidence and positive attitude you need to press on, tackle the areas you need the most help in, and ultimately do well on this test.

3. The Weakness Approach – Study the sections that you feel are your weakest and move on from there. For example, are your Math skills rusty? Then start with chapters 4 and 5 and study them carefully. Once you have shored up your weak areas, move on to your stronger areas, building your knowledge and confidence page by page.

4. The Blank Slate Approach – Unsure of your strengths or your weaknesses? Then start anywhere you like in the book and branch out from there. As you review each section, you'll soon get an idea of how much you know (or don't know) about a given topic. By committing to studying, you're gaining knowledge and belief in yourself.

In working through the book – regardless of your chosen study approach – you'll eventually get to the point where you feel ready to take a practice test. At that point, go to the online REA Study Center: *www.rea.com/studycenter*, take the free practice test, and see how well you score. (You can also take the online practice test before you begin studying to gauge your overall understanding of the topics tested on the TEAS.) Diagnostic feedback pinpoints your strengths and weaknesses and shows you where you need further review.

Study hard, and good luck on your test!

Daniel Greenberg

ABOUT OUR AUTHOR

Daniel Greenberg has been a writer in the educational field for more than 20 years, developing dozens of practical workbooks that make Science, Math, Grammar, Vocabulary, Reading Skills, History, and other subjects both fun and educational. Mr. Greenberg's op-eds and graphic art have appeared in *The Washington Post* and *The New York Times* as well as on BBC radio.

ACKNOWLEDGMENTS

We gratefully acknowledge Pam Weston, Publisher, for setting the quality standards for production integrity and managing the publication to completion; John Paul Cording, Vice President, Technology, for coordinating the design and development of the REA Study Center; Larry B. Kling, Vice President, Editorial, for his overall direction; Michael Reynolds, Managing Editor, for coordinating development of this edition; PreMediaGlobal for typesetting this edition; and Weymouth Design and Christine Saul, Senior Graphic Designer, for designing our cover.

ABOUT RESEARCH & EDUCATION ASSOCIATION

Founded in 1959, Research & Education Association (REA) is dedicated to publishing the finest and most effective educational materials — including study guides and test preps — for students in middle school, high school, college, graduate school, and beyond.

Today, REA's wide-ranging catalog is a leading resource for teachers, students, and professionals. Visit *www.rea.com* to see a complete listing of all our titles.

Taking the TEAS

1.1 THE TEAS: A SNAPSHOT

A. The Test of Essential Academic Skills (TEAS) is used to assess nursing program applicants in the United States. The TEAS features 170 test items, 20 of which are not scored, making a total of 150 scored items.

B. The total time for the test is 209 minutes, broken down into four sections—Reading Comprehension, Mathematics, Science, and English and Language Usage (see below).

C. The test is given in both paper/pencil and computerized form.

D. Breakdowns for the four major subject areas are as follows.

	Scored Items	Percent of Test	Percent of Section	Time (min)
Reading Comprehension	42	28	100	58
Paragraph	19	13	45	
Informational Source	23	15	55	
Mathematics	30	20	100	51
Operations	19	13	63	
Measurement	4	3	13	
Data	3	2	10	
Algebra	4	3	13	

(continued)

(*continued*)

	Scored Items	Percent of Test	Percent of Section	Time (min)
Science	48	32	100	66
Anatomy/Physiology	11	7	23	
Life Science	15	10	31	
Physical Science	14	9	29	
Scientific Reasoning	8	5	17	
English and Language Usage	30	20	100	34
Grammar and Vocabulary	15	10	50	
Spelling and Punctuation	9	6	30	
Structure	6	4	20	
Total	150	100		209

E. All test items are multiple-choice.

F. For the paper-based version of the test, bring two or more No. 2 pencils to the test center. For the computer-based test, bring pencils or pens for notes. Be sure to bring proper ID to your test location.

G. Allow a time window of 4 hours for the test.

H. Register for the test at: *www.atitesting.com*. The price for the test is $60; however, please be advised that prices may vary in different locations. Test times and locations will be provided when you register.

I. This book comes with a practice test at the online REA Study Center. You can obtain additional practice using the ATI test banks.

J. Passing scores for the test vary depending on the school to which you are applying. Typically, applicants must score at least 70% correct to gain entrance into nursing schools. Results for tests taken are provided within 5 to 7 days in the ATI account you create when you register for the test.

K. If you are not satisfied with your score, you may re-register and retake the TEAS after a waiting period of 45 days.

1.2 IS NURSING FOR YOU?

A. Before settling on choosing nursing as a career, ask yourself the following questions:

1. Are you a compassionate, empathetic, caring person?

2. How well do you deal with stress?

3. How good are you at following directions?

4. How comfortable are you with a job that presents new challenges every day rather than the security of knowing what you are going to do every day?

5. How comfortable are you working with and serving people of all kinds of ethnicities and backgrounds?

6. How comfortable are you in dealing with sickness, pain, and the end of life?

7. How squeamish are you with regard to the most basic and "messy" human functions, both physical and psychological?

8. Are you a good team player?

9. How comfortable are you in dealing with difficult and even abusive people?

10. How good are you at admitting mistakes, learning from mistakes, and forgiving mistakes in others?

11. How good are you at critical thinking? Are you comfortable in expressing your point of view even in the face of strong resistance?

12. How responsible, reliable, and punctual are you?

13. How comfortable are you in following orders and directions even when they may be flawed?

B. What kind of a nurse do you want to be?

1. Nursing degrees come in four categories:

   - An Associate's Degree in Nursing (ADN) is issued by 2-year schools.

   - A Bachelor's Degree in Nursing (BDN) is issued by a 4-year college or university.

   - A Master's Degree in Nursing (MSN) is obtained after completing a BDN and requires completing a graduate master's program.

   - A Doctorate in nursing is the highest degree obtainable and focuses on the most advanced and analytical aspects of the nursing profession.

2. Nursing levels include:

   - A Licensed Practical Nurse (LPN) or a Licensed Vocational Nurse (LVN) has completed only 1 year of post–high school nursing education.

   - A Registered Nurse (RN) must have at least an ADN and typically requires a BDN. RNs must also pass a licensing test to practice.

   - Advanced categories for nursing include such things as Nurse Practitioner (NP) or Clinical Nurse Specialist (CNS).

3. In becoming a nurse, you will need to choose:

   - Medical specialty: e.g., surgery, OB/GYN, gastroenterology, emergency

   - Where you work: e.g., hospital, clinic, doctor's office, school, military, private practice, hospice, government agency

   - Nursing specialties include nurse anesthetist, nurse midwife, nurse administrator, home health nurse, general duty nurse

1.3 GENERAL TEST-TAKING STRATEGY

A. Answer every question. You are not penalized for wrong answers. So make sure that you provide every question with an answer even if it is an uneducated guess.

B. Guess. An educated guess—when you have some idea about the correct answer—is a much better choice than an uneducated "wild" guess in which you are randomly choosing an answer.

1. With an "uneducated" guess in which your answer choice is random, your answer has a 25% chance of being correct.

2. If you can eliminate one wrong answer, your guess has a 33% chance of being correct.

3. If you can eliminate two wrong answers, your guess has a 50% chance of being correct.

C. Easy questions first. Don't worry about answering questions in order. Look for questions you know first. This allows you to move ahead on the test and then come back to the more difficult questions and give them more thought.

D. Mark the tough questions. If a question is troublesome, ambiguous, or for some reason too hard to answer, circle it and come back to it later. If you have an answer but you're unsure of it, mark the question and revisit it later.

E. Watch the clock. Follow the percentages (see pages 1–2) for each test section. Aim to have spare time after you have gone through the entire test.

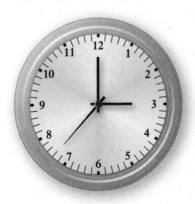

F. For example, after 15 minutes in the 58-minute (roughly 1 hour) Reading Comprehension test, you should have completed well over 25% of the test items, having answered at least 10 but preferably 12 or more of the 42 test items.

G. After about a half hour in the Reading Comprehension section, your test should be more than half complete, having finished a minimum of 20 and preferably around 25 of the 42 questions.

H. Your goal should be to complete the test with about 10 minutes to spare. This will give you time to go over the "straggler" questions that you couldn't initially answer or to reconsider tough questions.

I. If you don't reach your goal of having spare time at the end of the test, don't worry. The most important time management element is to stay calm and work steadily.

J. **Be intuitive.** In general, your first stab at a question you don't know is often your best. If an answer *seems* better, it often is.

K. **Identify what is being asked.** Your first order of business for a question is to make sure that you are answering what is actually being asked for. For example, look at the units of the answer for gas mileage. If your answer is not in miles per gallon, it can't be correct.

L. **Watch out for decoy answers.** Most questions have one or two wrong answers that are way off the mark and at least one answer that is plausible in some way.

    1. Eliminate the clearly wrong answers right away.

    2. Then consider the two or three plausible answers remaining. Try plugging these answers back into the question to see if they make sense.

    3. If you still can't identify the best answer, use your intuition to make an educated guess.

M. Review your answer. A good strategy is to work as quickly as possible but always take the time to review the answer that you obtain. Ask yourself:

1. Does this answer make sense?

2. Am I falling for a decoy?

3. Did I find the answer that the problem was actually asking for?

N. Be cool. Stressing out over the test makes your results worse, not better. So focus on serenity. Think of your stress as an energy source that can be harnessed and used in a positive rather than a negative way.

O. Dumb Mistakes That People Make When Taking the Test

1. **Failing to eat a good breakfast.** Your brain needs to be in top shape during the test. You can't afford to run out of focus or energy. So try to eat well and sleep well as you prepare for the test.

2. **Overconfidence.** If you are a qualified applicant, the TEAS should not seem overly difficult. However, you shouldn't take the test lightly either. Be serious. Give the test the respect it deserves. Your future may depend on it.

3. **A bad attitude.** You may consider yourself a poor test taker, but apprehension, fear, and pessimism can only make your performance worse. Assume an air of quiet confidence.

4. **Cramming.** You may be able to cram for a narrowly focused junior high spelling test, but the TEAS is too broad, too varied, and too general to be crammed for. Cramming can only result in making you tired and anxious on exam day.

P. Smart Tips That Help People When Taking the Test

1. **Exercise.** Exercise does more than build physical stamina; it also builds mental stamina. In fact, you will need plenty of both kinds of stamina for taking the test. So get into an exercise routine weeks and months before you take the test. You will eat better, sleep better, and study better as a result of it.

2. **Get help.** Don't know much about chemistry? Rather than try to learn it all on your own, seek out someone who can help—a friend, sibling, teacher, tutor, or parent.

3. **Set goals.** The key to getting things done is to map out your study goals ahead of time. Chart your progress on a table or graph.

4. **Be honest with yourself.** If you're not good with fractions, it won't help to skip over them and hope they don't show up on the test. Realistically assess your strengths and weaknesses. Work extra hard on the places where you need help.

1.4 SETTING UP A STUDY PLAN

A. First, determine how much time you have before the test and how much time you can realistically devote toward preparation each day. Do you have months? Weeks? Only a few days? The answer to these questions will determine how your study plan proceeds.

B. Find your strengths and weaknesses. This is precisely where taking our online practice test may come in handy. Then find those topics in this book and work on them. For example,

	Strength or Weakness?	Priority (1–5)	Date Studied	Time (min)
Reading Comprehension				
Reading skills				
Printed documents				
Directions				
Comparison				
Mathematics				
Basic operations				
Rounding and place value				
Estimating and mental math				
Integers and negative numbers				
Fractions				
Decimals and percentages				

(continued)

(*continued*)

	Strength or Weakness?	Priority (1–5)	Date Studied	Time (min)
Expressions and equations				
Ratios and proportions				
Measurement and conversion				
Data and graphs				
Other topics				
Science				
Cells				
Body systems				
Biochemistry				
Genetics and DNA				
Ecology and evolution				
Scientific reasoning				
Atoms and molecules				
Chemical reactions				
Phases and solutions				
Motion				
Newton's laws and gravity				
Force, energy, and work				
Electricity				
English and Language Usage				
Parts of speech				
Sentences				
Punctuation				
Spelling and vocabulary				
Grammar errors				
Total	150	100%		209

testing might reveal that you have deficient knowledge in body systems, such as how the circulatory, digestive, and other systems function in the human body. If this is a trouble area for you, go to the Body Systems section in this book and get to work.

C. Set up a calendar on which you schedule various study areas and mark off how much time you spend on them in the table above.

D. An alternative strategy, especially if you have a lot of time, involves working systematically through this entire book from start to finish or chapter by chapter. You should find the review to be extremely helpful, and you will be surprised at how many *new* things you learn even in areas in which you previously thought you were strong.

E. Use triage at all times. If you have only a few weeks to prepare, you need to focus only on weaknesses and general areas. You don't have time to be systematic. On the other hand, if your time is not limited and you find that spending extra time on a topic such as chemistry is valuable, go ahead and do it.

F. Be steady. Have a regular study time and try not to let "real life" interfere with it. Remember, the work you put in now for this test has the promise of paying off over an entire lifetime.

1.5 TEST STRATEGIES FOR SPECIFIC QUESTION TYPES

A. Reading Comprehension Passages

One of the common question types on the TEAS is the long reading passage from which you'll need to draw conclusions and make judgments.

1. Read the title and scan the paragraphs. Get a feel for what the topic is and what to expect from your reading. Note whether multiple questions are associated with the passage; in most cases, they will be.

2. After previewing the title and the general text structure, many expert test takers like to go over the questions *before* they read the passage. Note: This technique may or may not be for you! However, if you are one of those people who benefits from a question preview, go ahead and do it.

3. Read quickly but carefully. After each section, briefly review what you just read before you go on. After finishing, consider the piece as a whole. How did the paragraphs fit together? What was the main point of the piece? How was it supported?

4. Feel free to underline, circle, and write notes as you read. For example, if you view a sentence as providing critical support for a key idea within the passage, mark it clearly.

5. Finish the passage and go on to the questions. If the first question or two seem daunting, keep moving until you come to a question you are sure of. Then go back to the more difficult questions.

B. Math Word Problems and Problem Solving

The TEAS Math section has many different types of word problems. Some are simple and require just a quick calculation. Others are complex and may require a detailed analysis. For any word problem, whether it involves whole numbers, fractions, algebra, or any of the topics in Chapters 4 or 5, follow these basic steps.

PROBLEM SOLVING: BASIC STEPS

1. **Read the problem carefully.** Many problems are misunderstood simply because the problem solver fails to understand the situation.

2. **If possible, solve immediately.** If you see the key relationship right away, there is no need to go through a complex analysis. Solve. Then go on to step 7 below.

3. **Underline, circle, write, list.** If you don't see the key relationship right away, mark up the problem by circling, underlining, or making lists and writing equations. You

may wish to list information in two sections that roughly constitute "What I know" and "What I don't know."

4. **Identify what you need to find.** This is usually the most important step in the process. Find out what you need to know. Focus on the units of your unknown such as inches, grams, boxes, milliliters, or miles per hour.

5. **Make a plan.** For simple problems, this might entail nothing more than identifying an operation—addition, subtraction, multiplication, or division—to carry out. For more complex problems, your plan may involve more than one step and more than one operation. In your plan, look for **key words**.

Add +	Subtract −	Multiply ×	Divide ÷
in all sum	less than	product of	quotient per
total	fewer than	times	each equal
together	more than	multiplied	parts split
sum total	minus	by increased	divided by
combined	difference	by a factor of	ratio of
plus	take away	total in all	
	left over		
	decreased by		
	increased by		

6. **Set up the problem and solve.** Carry out your plan and get an answer.

7. **Go over your answer.** First ask, "Did I find what I was looking for?" If you were looking for miles per gallon and you found gallons per mile, your answer is probably wrong. Check your units. Check your computations. Make sure that your answer solves the problem.

C. Problem Solving Do's and Don'ts

 DO

- **Write.** Writing things out helps you visualize the problem. Also draw, diagram, model—do anything that helps you see relationships.

- **Estimate.** Use estimation both before and after you solve the problem. Preview to estimate what your answer should be; then check to see if your answer was correct.

- **Ask yourself, "Does this make sense?"** This is probably the most important step after you've solved the problem. Does your final answer fit the situation and seem reasonable for the context of the problem? If not, it's probably best to rethink the problem.

- **Think simple.** The test is not out to force you to make complicated and "messy" calculations. If you get an answer that seems overly messy looking or complicated, it's probably wrong.

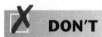

DON'T

- **Try to do it in your head.** Mental math and estimation work only with simple relationships and simple numbers. If you have any doubt, write out the problem. Being able to see your thought process on paper is always a good check.

- **Jump to conclusions.** Make sure you understand what the problem is asking for before you answer it.

- **Rush.** The worst thing about rushing is that it makes you sloppy and slapdash. Work fast and keep moving but always focus on staying calm and steady.

- **Be stubborn.** Being sure you're right is good. Being *too* sure is not good. If your problem-solving procedure or your answer seems suspect, don't hesitate to rethink the problem and start all over.

D. Grammar Question Type: Which Sentence Is Written Correctly?

One of the most common—and most important—question types in the Language section of the TEAS is a variation of "Which sentence is written correctly?"

1. **Look for obvious mistakes.** Questions might include such errors as failing to capitalize the first word in the sentence, misplaced apostrophes, or failing to put punctuation at the end of the sentence.

2. **Is the sentence complete?** Answer choices may feature dependent clauses or other nonsentences trying to pass as sentences. Make sure that the sentence has a complete subject and complete predicate and is not a dependent clause. For example:

   After the rain stopped in the meadow. (Not a complete sentence)

   After the rain stopped in the meadow, we ate lunch. (Complete sentence)

3. **Do the subject and verb agree?** Examples:

   Is Mary and John interested in lunch? (Incorrect)

   Are Mary and John interested in lunch? (Correct)

4. **Are there pronoun or possessive errors?** Objective and subjective cases should not be confused.

   Bob gave advice to Mary and I. (Incorrect)

   Bob gave advice to Mary and me. (Correct)

   Everyone should keep their room clean. (Incorrect)

   Everyone should keep his or her room clean. (Correct)

5. **Should the sentence be broken up?** Test questions often feature run-on sentences that should be broken into two sentences:

   Bob is hungry Mary is not hungry. (Incorrect)

   Bob is hungry. Mary is not hungry. (Correct)

6. **Are there comma errors?** Comma errors include commas in a series; comma splices, which incorrectly join two independent clauses; and failure to insert commas with coordinating conjunctions and dependent clauses.

   Bob is hungry, Mary is nervous. (Incorrect; comma splice)

   Bob is hungry. Mary is nervous. (Correct)

   John ate rice beans and salsa. (Incorrect)

   John ate rice, beans, and salsa. (Correct)

   Bob was hungry so Mary gave him a bagel. (Incorrect)

   Bob was hungry, so Mary gave him a bagel. (Correct)

After dinner we went for a walk. (Incorrect)

After dinner, we went for a walk. (Correct)

7. **Are there spelling errors?** Look for commonly confused words, such as *effect* and *affect* or *accept* and *except*.

8. **Is the sentence unclear or ambiguous?** Focus on making sure that the sentence communicates what it intends to communicate.

Evita wore her yellow dress on the beach that was breathtakingly beautiful. (Unclear: What was breathtakingly beautiful, the dress or the beach?)

On a breathtakingly beautiful beach, Evita wore her yellow dress. (Clear)

E. **Science Graphics**

The Science sections of the TEAS contain a large number of graphs, charts, and other types of visual images. To interpret these items, follow the steps below.

1. **Identification.** Many TEAS science questions are not asking for analysis; they are simply asking you to identify a familiar graphic. For example, the test might ask you to identify a food web or a DNA diagram. In this case, you simply match the name of the graphic to the graphic itself.

2. **Trends.** A graph question may ask you to identify trends within the graph. For example, a graph may compare solubility of two different substances in water as the temperature rises. Your task is to identify the trend (increasing? decreasing? variable?) for each substance.

   a. With graphs, look for relationships. Make sure you identify each axis of the graph and understand what the graph is showing.

   b. With tables you often need to look for trends within the data. Are quantities increasing or decreasing? How does one data category compare with others?

3. **Drawing conclusions vs. extracting data.** Make sure you understand what the question is asking for.

a. Many graphic questions ask you to draw a conclusion: Which is greater? What change do you see?

b. Other questions require you to extract information: Find the atomic weight of chlorine. Which heart chamber pumps the blood to the lungs?

4. **Diagrams.** Many graphics are abstract diagrams that show relationships and trends. A Venn diagram, for example, might compare prokaryotes and eukaryotes. A carbon-cycle diagram might show the forms that carbon takes as it progresses through the environment.

5. **Schematics.** Some diagrams depict relationships between actual items. A circuit diagram, for example, shows how electrical elements are wired. A mitosis diagram shows each step in the process of cell division.

Reading Comprehension

2.1 **READING SKILLS**

A. Main Idea Skills: Overview

   1. The **main idea** identifies the reason for a text to be written.

   2. The **topic** of a text is what the text is generally about.

   3. Thus, the topic of an article might be dogs, but the main idea of the same text might be that beagles are the dogs with the keenest sense of smell.

   4. Although the entire text has a main idea, each paragraph within a text also has its own main idea.

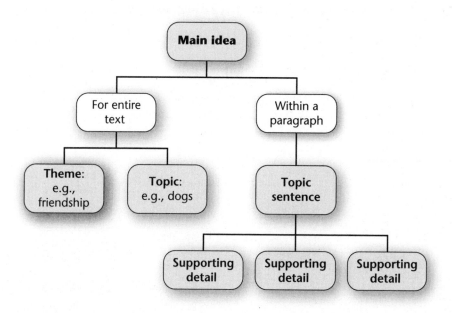

5. Within a paragraph, each main idea is introduced by a **topic sentence**, typically followed by **supporting details** that work to provide evidence for the main idea. The topic sentence is usually the first sentence in a paragraph.

6. A **theme** refers to a text's highest and most general subject. Themes are typically "big" ideas such as love, beauty, or the meaning of friendship.

☞ For exercises involving **main idea** and other topics, **see sections 2.1 G and 2.1 H.**

B. Author's Purpose: Overview

1. Authors generally have one of four purposes for writing: to **explain**, to **persuade**, to **entertain**, or to **express feelings**.

2. **Example:** A description of how different dog breeds are classified
   - **Author's purpose: To explain:** Provides information

3. **Example:** A blog post that tells you that you should buy *locally grown food*
   - **Author's purpose: To persuade:** Attempts to convince you of something, that *beagles are the best dog breed.*

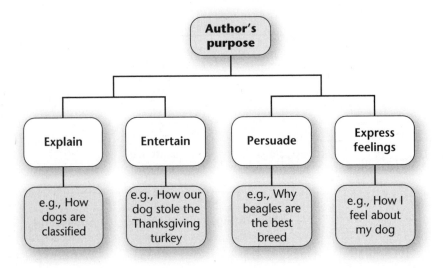

4. **Example:** A hilarious account of how our dog ran off with our Thanksgiving turkey

   • **Author's purpose: To entertain:** The account of the dog aims to amuse and delight.

5. **Example:** A poem about my dog

   • **Author's purpose: To express feelings:** The poem intends to express my feelings about my dog.

For exercises involving an **author's purpose** and other topics, **see section 2.1 H.**

C. Facts, Opinions, Biases, Stereotypes: Overview

1. An **opinion** is a statement that reflects a person's personal judgment, which may or may not be supported by evidence or facts.

2. **Facts** are statements that can be documented, verified, and supported by evidence.

3. **Example:** Wednesday is the best day of the week.

   • **Opinion:** This is an opinion because it cannot be proven or verified that Wednesday is the best day of the week.

4. **Example:** Congress passed the law on October 3.

   • **Fact:** This is a fact because it can be verified by, for example, a newspaper article or the official Congressional record.

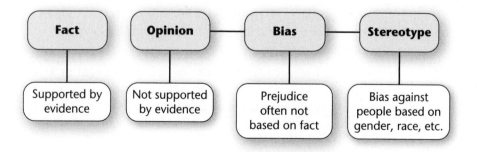

Fact	Opinion	Bias	Stereotype
Supported by evidence	Not supported by evidence	Prejudice often not based on fact	Bias against people based on gender, race, etc.

5. A **bias** is a prejudice that is typically based on a faulty opinion. Having a bias predisposes a person to seeing a situation in a certain way and drawing certain conclusions.

6. **Stereotypes** are biases about people, typically based on their ethnicity, gender, age, skin color, and so on.

7. **Example:** Ralph won't buy American-made cars because he thinks they are cheaply made. If you ask him for evidence that they are cheaply made, he can't supply it.

   - **Bias:** Ralph has a slanted view that is not based on evidence.

8. **Example:** Cheryl thinks Mark is a bad driver because he's Asian.

   - **Stereotype:** Cheryl is not basing her view on facts but on a false view of an ethnic group.

 For exercises involving **facts, opinions**, and other topics, **see section 2.1 H.**

D. Text Structure: Overview

1. The structure or look of a text can make the text easier to read. Text structure can also provide clues to the reader about the meaning of the text.

2. A **sequence** text structure can take the form of a list, numbered steps, a bulleted list, or a series in outline form.

3. **Problem-solution** text structure introduces a problem in one paragraph or section and then goes on to provide a solution for that problem in the next paragraph or section.

   - **Example:** The first paragraph describes a problem that local landfills are overfilled. The paragraph that follows describes a recycling program that aims to solve the problem.

4. **Cause-and-effect** text structure describes an event or a phenomenon in one paragraph or section and then goes on to show the consequence or *effect* of that event in the next paragraph or section.

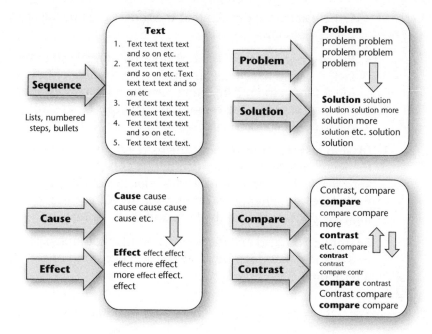

- **Example:** The first paragraph describes a tsunami. The paragraph that follows describes the damage done by the tsunami.

5. **Compare and contrast** shows both similarities and differences between items.

   - **Example:** A paragraph describes how two cell phone models are similar and different.

For exercises involving **text structure** and other topics, **see section 2.1 H.**

E. Conclusions, Inferences, Predictions: Overview

1. Drawing a **conclusion** involves taking facts in a text and extending them logically to deduce important ideas and other forms of information.

2. **Example:** A book about the history of the Vietnam War states that the war lasted from 1964 to 1975. The same book profiles a soldier who joined the military in 1978 at 19 years of age.

- **Conclusion:** You deduce that the soldier did not see combat in Vietnam.

- **Reasoning:** Although the text does not directly state this fact, it would have been impossible for the solider to have fought in Vietnam if he didn't join the military until after the war was over and he was only 19 years of age. You have drawn a logical conclusion from the text.

3. Making an **inference** requires the reader to "read between the lines" of a text and use such things as facts, prior knowledge, common sense, and tendencies of the author to deduce something that is not explicitly stated yet seems logically consistent with the facts and their context.

4. **Example:** You read an article about events that took place in a hospital that describes a snowstorm occurring one afternoon.

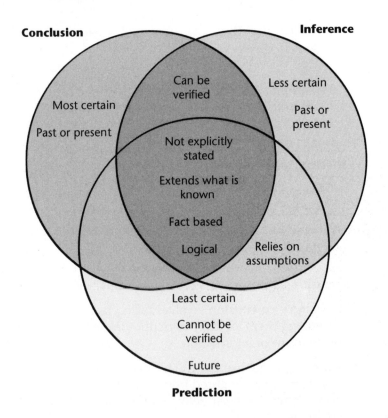

- **Inference:** You make the assumption that the events took place during a winter month.

- **Reasoning:** Having snow on the ground typically indicates that events are taking place in December, January, or February.

- **Active reading:** Inferences can turn out to be right or wrong. After you make an inference, keep looking for additional clues as you read to confirm (or disprove) your inference.

5. Making a **prediction** requires the reader to extend beyond the text and deduce something that will occur in the future.

6. **Example:** In a story about an unconventional teacher, the teacher uses computer games to try to motivate a troubled student.

- **Prediction:** Based on the context of the story, you predict that the student will become a computer "whiz" and earn a scholarship to college.

- **Reasoning:** You figure that if the author spends time describing this unconventional teaching method, it must be a method that ultimately pays off in success.

- **Active reading:** Similar to inferences, predictions may or may not turn out to be correct. The important thing is to use your prediction to process information as you read. In this case, you are keeping your eye on the troubled student to see how that student fares in the future. If your prediction turns out to be wrong, it has still been useful in helping you understand the story.

 For exercises involving **drawing conclusions, making inferences, and making predictions, see sections 2.1 G and 2.2 H**.

F. Types of Texts: Overview

1. Texts generally have one of four basic forms:

   a. A **narrative** tells a story or relates a sequence of events.

   b. An **expository** text explains or describes something.

   c. **Technical** writing provides highly detailed information on a topic.

   d. **Persuasive** writing attempts to build a case for a point of view and sway the views of the reader.

2. **Narrative examples:** *To Kill a Mockingbird*, what you did on your vacation, *Star Wars*, Ben Franklin's autobiography

   • **Reason:** All of these examples tell a story or sequence of events.

3. **Expository text examples:** Advice on how to improve your finances, a description of the British royal wedding, an explanation of how Obamacare will affect you

   • **Reason:** All of these examples explain.

4. **Persuasive writing examples:** Endorsement of a political candidate, essay to convince you to vote, newspaper column that asks you to take action against global climate change

   • **Reason:** All of these examples try to persuade.

5. **Technical writing examples:** Instructions for a new tablet computer, specifications for high-tech machinery, protocol for a scientific procedure

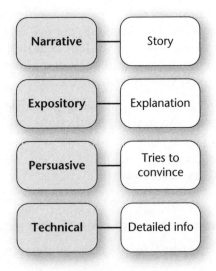

- **Reason:** All of these examples provide highly technical information in detail.

 For exercises involving different **types of informational text** and other topics, **see sections 2.2 A and 2.2 B**.

G. Passage 1: Problems

The following five questions refer to the passage that follows. These questions cover **theme**, **inference**, **supporting detail**, **summarizing**, and inferring the meaning of words in **context**.

On March 6, 1770, John Adams was awoken with a banging on his door. The man at the door, Mr. James Forrest, a wealthy Boston merchant, had a desperate request. Would Adams represent Forrest's friends in court? Adams balked. Although he would go on to be one of our nation's Founding Fathers and its second president, Adams at the time was just a struggling young Boston lawyer. Weren't there more prominent attorneys in town for the chore?

However, as Adams soon learned, these were no ordinary clients. They were the British soldiers who had been accused of murdering five citizens in the notorious Boston Massacre a day earlier. Newspaper headlines were already decrying them as MONSTERS! As Adams soon learned, Forrest had already been to just about every lawyer in Boston. Adams was the soldiers' last chance. Would he take the case?

At this point, Adams might have taken the easy way out. He might have explained that his cousin and close friend Sam Adams was the leader of the secret anti-British revolutionary group known as the Sons of Liberty. He might have told Forrest that although he was not an official member of the group, he had attended its meetings and strongly sympathized with its cause.

He might have explained that defending the British soldiers would not simply ruin his reputation as a lawyer and a revolutionary patriot, but it might also threaten his life. Emotions since the event had brought Boston to a boil. Rather than looking forward to a fair trial for the soldiers, most citizens wanted them punished and were likely to resent anyone who tried to help them.

And yet, with all of these reasons to say no, Adams ended up saying yes. He took the case. When asked later what his reasons were, Adams gave the famous reply, "I'd rather see five guilty people go free than one innocent person suffer unfairly." This attitude of putting justice ahead of partisanship and cool judgment and fairness ahead of prejudice and hot emotion would serve Adams—and the new nation—well in the years to come.

2.1

Problem 1:

Which of the following identifies the theme of the passage?

A) Justice   B) The Boston Massacre   C) John Adams   D) Revenge

STRATEGY

The **theme** refers to a text's highest and most general subject. Themes are typically "big" ideas such as love, the importance of family, beauty, and the meaning of friendship. Look for an answer choice that identifies the "big" idea in the text.

THINK

- What is the overarching "big" idea that this passage expresses?

- The Boston Massacre (B) and John Adams (C) qualify more as topics than themes. They focus on the subject matter rather than the major, overarching ideas in the text, so they are not correct responses.

- Revenge (D) qualifies as a theme, but there is nothing in the passage that suggests revenge as a major idea.

- This leaves justice (A) as the correct answer choice. Justice is a big idea, and it accurately reflects the central idea in the text.

2.1

Problem 2:

What can you conclude about John Adams from the text?

A) He thought that the soldiers were guilty.

B) He thought that the soldiers were innocent.

C) He was fair-minded.

D) He had many friends who were British.

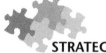

STRATEGY

Making an **inference** requires the reader to "read between the lines" of a text and deduce something that is not explicitly stated yet seems logically consistent with the facts in the text and its context.

THINK

- Which of the answer choice statements are supported either directly or indirectly by information in the passage?

- There is no indication in the text that Adams believed that the soldiers were either innocent or guilty, so both (A) and (B) are incorrect. The fact that he takes the case implies only that he wants to see the soldiers treated fairly.

- There is no indication in the text of how Adams feels about the British. He is a sympathizer with his cousin Sam but has not officially become a revolutionary, perhaps because he has sympathy for the British as well.

- What does come clearly from the text is that Adams is concerned with fairness. He may think that the soldiers are guilty and monstrous. Nevertheless, it is clear from his statement, "I'd rather see five guilty people go free than one innocent person suffer unfairly" that fairness is important to him, making (C) the correct response.

2.1

Problem 3:

Which detail best supports a position that Adams did NOT take the case out of a sense of justice?

A) Boston is described as "boiling over."

B) Adams is described as a "struggling" lawyer.

C) The text states that Adams's reputation as a lawyer is at risk.

D) The text states that Adams's life is at risk.

STRATEGY

A **supporting detail** refers to a statement or fact within the text that supports a main idea in the text. Supporting details can be used to justify conclusions that readers draw or **inferences** that they make.

THINK

- Suppose Adams took the case not out of a sense of responsibility or justice but for some other reason. Which detail in the passage would best support this view?

- Boston "boiling over" (A) and Adams risking his reputation (C) or life (D) all support the idea that Adams does not take the case for some venal reason but is taking it because he believes all people, even "murderous" British soldiers, should be treated justly.

- The fact that Adams is described as a "struggling" lawyer would provide support for the idea that he took the case for money rather than justice. A struggling lawyer needs money. Had Adams already been one of Boston's more "prominent" lawyers, one would assume that he would be less likely to take a case purely for money. That said, the rest of the text does not support this conclusion. The correct answer choice is (B).

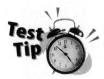

Note that the question is hypothetical. It is not claiming that Adams actually took the case for some mercenary reason, but rather, if justice had not been his motive, which piece of evidence would best support that hypothetical position?

2.1

Problem 4:

Which of the following statements best summarizes Adams's quote that, "I'd rather see five guilty people go free than one innocent person suffer unfairly"?

A) Accuracy is more important than justice.

B) Justice and accuracy are equally important.

C) Accuracy is at least three times more important than justice.

D) Justice is more important than accuracy.

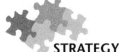

STRATEGY

Summarizing requires a reader to distill and condense a text into its most basic form, stripping away all inessential items and leaving just the most critical information. In this case, you need to interpret the statement in light of its context and its meaning within the entire passage.

THINK

- What does the quote really mean? Which of the answer choice statements best captures the essence of the quote and restates its primary point?

- Answer choices (A), (B), and (C) all focus on accuracy rather than justice. These choices would match a statement that claimed the opposite of what Adams was actually claiming. The view of Adams was that the greatest mistake of all is to punish an innocent person. Although it is wrong to let guilty people go free, he would rather see that occur than have a single person be condemned without cause.

- Answer choice (D) is a good condensation of Adams's view and the correct response. He would rather see crimes go unpunished than see innocent people prosecuted unfairly.

2.1

Problem 5:

In the context of this text, the word *prominent* means

A) outspoken.   B) well known and successful.

C) expensive.   D) reputable and conventional.

STRATEGY

Words can change meaning based on how they are used in the **context**, or exact circumstances in a text. To identify this meaning, take everything into account, including how and where the word is used in the sentence, what it means to the paragraph and the overall text, and what you infer as the author's purpose and his or her goals in writing the text.

THINK

- How is the word *prominent* being used in this context?
- *Prominent* refers to someone or something that stands out from its background as important. In another context, *prominent* could reasonably be taken in to mean outspoken (A), reputable (D), or even expensive (C).

- However, in this context, it is clear that the author is trying to highlight the fact that Adams is still trying to establish his reputation as a lawyer at the time of the Boston Massacre, so more *prominent* lawyers would be those who were more well known and successful than him, making (B) the correct response.

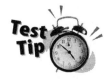

When the definition of a word in context is asked for, pay special attention to how the word is being used in the sentence. Is the word functioning as a noun? A verb? An adjective or adverb? Does the standard or conventional definition of the word apply in this situation, or is the word being used in some special way in which its connotations differ from the standard meaning?

H. Passage 2: Problems

The following five questions refer to the passage that follows. They cover **author's purpose**, **main idea**, **topic sentences**, **text structure**, and **fact vs. opinion**.

Although I personally do not drink soda and strictly limit its consumption for my children, I nevertheless must speak here in opposition to the mayor's ban on soft drinks larger than 16 ounces being sold in our city.

No one disputes the idea that our society is suffering from an obesity epidemic. Rates of obesity and being overweight are skyrocketing among children in our country. In the United States, about two-thirds of adults now qualify as being either obese or overweight.

This trend has enormous consequences, threatening the health and reducing the lifespan of hundreds of millions of Americans. Obesity is linked to a number of different ailments, including diabetes and heart disease, and economically it is a major cause of the health care crisis in the United States.

The case against sugary sodas is not quite so clear-cut, but it is convincing nevertheless. There is no doubt that excess consumption of sugar, especially in liquid form, is a major contributor to obesity. There is also little doubt that if soda consumption were reduced, then obesity rates would also be likely to decline.

However, as bad as soda is for people, I see no principle either in our legal tradition or our general cultural mores to ban its consumption. Last I looked, freedom was the most important principle in American life. We are first and foremost a free people who cherish our freedoms—including the freedom to make foolish decisions.

Is it good for you to drink soda? No, but I'll defend your right to do it. And that's why I oppose the mayor's ban on large sodas—because it's against freedom.

2.1

Problem 6:

What appears to be the author's purpose in writing this piece?

A) To provide facts and figures about obesity

B) To explain why soda is not harmful

C) To advocate against a ban on sodas

D) To amuse the audience

STRATEGY

Authors generally have one of four purposes for writing: to **explain**, to **persuade**, to **entertain**, or to **express feelings**.

THINK

- What is the author trying to accomplish here? Does the author want to make a point? Then he or she is likely to be explaining or persuading. On the other hand, if the author is primarily trying to engage the reader's emotions, then he or she is trying to entertain or express feelings.

- Although the piece is entertaining to a degree and provides a great deal of information about obesity and soda, entertainment and providing information are secondary purposes for the author, making (A) and (D) incorrect choices. Answer choice (B) is incorrect because the piece argues that soda *is* harmful, not that it's not harmful.

- The primary purpose of the author is clearly to persuade. At the beginning and end the author states his or her position: the author is against the soda ban on the grounds that it limits freedom, making (C) the correct response.

2.1

Problem 7:

Which of the following is a topic sentence in the passage?

A) There is no doubt that excess consumption of sugar, especially in liquid form, is a major contributor to obesity.

B) Although I personally do not drink soda and strictly limit its consumption for my children, I nevertheless must speak here in opposition to the mayor's ban on soft drinks larger than 16 ounces being sold in our city.

C) Rates of obesity and being overweight are skyrocketing among children in our country.

D) Last I looked, freedom was the most important principle in American life.

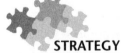

STRATEGY

The **topic sentence** in a paragraph or larger text is the sentence that identifies the **main idea** of the text. Typically, the topic sentence appears first in a paragraph and is followed by a series of supporting details.

THINK

- What is the main idea of this passage, and which sentence expresses that idea? Which sentence expresses this main idea?

- Look for a sentence that comes first in a paragraph—it is likely to be a topic sentence. (A) and (C) provide key information about obesity, but they do not get at the main idea of the passage, which is to take a position against the soda ban. Only (B) expresses this main idea, so it is the correct response.

2.1

Problem 8:

Which kind of text structure is illustrated by paragraphs 2 and 3 of the text?

A) Sequence   B) Problem–solution

C) Comparison–contrast   D) Cause and effect

STRATEGY

The most common **text structures** are **sequence, problem–solution, cause and effect,** or **comparison–contrast.**

THINK

- Which text structure model fits these paragraphs best?

- Paragraph 2 describes the extent of the obesity epidemic with respect to both adults and children. Paragraph 3 identifies the consequences of these trends, which are major health and economic problems.

- Clearly, this structure of first providing facts and second showing the consequences or results of those facts fits a cause-and-effect pattern. The causes are the skyrocketing obesity rates. The effects are the outcomes of those sky-rocketing rates. This makes answer choice (D) the correct response.

2.1

Problem 9:

Cultural mores

A) are informal moral or ethical standards.

B) celebrate ethnic customs and traditions.

C) reflect unconscious prejudices and biases.

D) exist only among the middle classes.

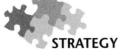

STRATEGY

Examine how the word is being used in the **context** of the sentence and how it fits in with the entire passage.

THINK

- How is the term *cultural mores* used in the text? What clues does the text provide that help define this term?

- Cultural mores may refer to customs and traditions, but clearly in this context, they have nothing to do with ethnicity, so (B) is incorrect. Similarly, cultural mores may reflect unconscious attitudes (C), but within this situation, they are neither biased nor prejudiced.

- (A) is the correct response because in this context, cultural mores refer to generalized standards that all segments of American society seem to agree on. (D) is incorrect because all segments of society, not just the middle classes, have cultural mores.

2.1

Problem 10:

Which sentence from this passage expresses an opinion?

A) Rates of obesity and being overweight are skyrocketing among children in our country.

B) In the United States, for example, about two-thirds of adults now qualify as being either obese or overweight.

C) There is no doubt that excess consumption of sugar, especially in liquid form, is a major contributor to obesity.

D) Is it good for you to drink soda? No, but I'll defend your right to do it.

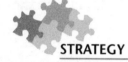

STRATEGY

An **opinion** is a statement that reflects a person's personal judgment, which may or may not be supported by **facts**, which are statements that can be documented and supported by evidence.

THINK

- Which of the sentences states a personal judgment that would be difficult to verify or prove?

- (A), (B), and (C) all state verifiable facts. You could document the rates of obesity among children (A) and adults (B) and that consumption of sugar in liquid form is harmful (C).

- More problematic would be to prove that people are foolish to drink soda. After all, although millions of people who drink soda are overweight or obese, millions more are perfectly healthy and would be likely to resent being labeled as "foolish," making (D) the correct answer choice.

2.2 PRINTED DOCUMENTS

A. Types: Overview

1. **Browse:** A label, bill, or form should not be read in a comprehensive order from beginning to end as you would read a narrative. Instead, browse. Focus first on what catches your eye and then zoom in on the details.

2. **Scan:** Scan labels, bills, and forms for specific information. On an ingredients list, you might want to scan to see how many grams of fat a food contains. On a form or bill, you might want to see if there is a request for any kind of action or payment.

3. **Use position:** The position of text on a form, bill, or label is often critical. General identification information is usually at the top of the text. More detailed and specialized information is positioned lower down. Many documents have specific locations for standard information. To find the account number for a bill, for example, always look in the upper right-hand corner of the first page.

4. **Use logic:** A bill may tell you when your last payment was but not how much it was. However, you can determine the amount of that payment by subtracting the previous balance from the balance at the beginning of the billing period.

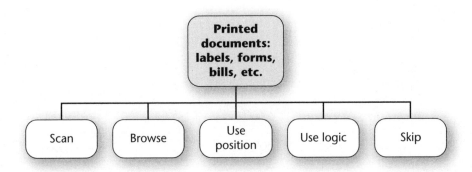

5. **Skip:** Usually, you do not want to read everything in a label, form, or bill. Some paragraphs contain technical or irrelevant information that has no value to you, so skip over them.

B. Forms and Bills: Problems

The following questions refer to the document shown. They pertain to reading a document like the one shown here.

Department of Treasury
Internal Revenue Service
PO BOX 249
Memphis, TN 38101-0249

Notice	CP14
Tax Year	2007
Notice date	March 2, 2012
Social Security number	XXX-XX-XXXX
To contact us	Phone 1-XXX-XXX-XXXX
Your Caller ID	1234
Page 1 of 4	
Record Locator:	PL142578194004

LISH, RALPH A
STEINER, LISA C
46 ABERFOYLE RD
NEW ROCHELLE, NY 10804

You have unpaid taxes for 2012
Amount due: $537.40

Our records show you have unpaid taxes for the tax year ending on December 31, 2013 (Form 1040).

Billing Summary

Tax you owed	53,183.00
Payments and credits	–3,328.00
Failure-to-file penalty	286.47
Failure-to-pay penalty	127.32
Failure-to-pay proper estimated tax penalty	145.00
Interest charges	123.61
Amount due by March 23, 2013	**$537.40**

What you need to do immediately

Pay immediately
• Send us the amount due of $537.40 by March 23, 2013 to avoid additional penalty and interest charges.

Continued on back...

Lish, Ralph A, Steiner, Lisa C
46 Aberfoyle Rd
New Rochelle, NY 10804

Notice	CP14
Notice date	March 2, 2012
Social Security Number	XXX-XX-XXXX

Payment

• Make your check or money order payable to the United States Treasury.
• Write your Social Security number (XXX-XX-XXXX), the tax year (2007), and the form number (104D) on your payment and any correspondence.

Amount due by
March 23, 2013

$537.40

INTERNAL REVENUE SERVICE
CINCINNATI, OH 45999-0150
s018999546711s

2.2

Problem 1:

Who is the document from?

A) Internal Revenue Service (IRS)

B) New York State Tax Department

C) City of Los Angeles

D) New York State legislature

STRATEGY

Scan the document for identification information. Then draw conclusions.

THINK

- The top of the document or letterhead usually identifies the sender. It is clear that this document is from the IRS.

- This document cannot be from any state or city agency because it is clearly from the federal IRS. This makes (A) the correct response.

2.2

Problem 2:

What is the purpose of the document?

A) It is informing the taxpayers that they overpaid their taxes and will be getting a refund.

B) It is informing the taxpayers that they overpaid their taxes and will not be getting a refund.

C) It is informing the taxpayers that they overpaid their taxes and they owe money.

D) It is informing the taxpayers that they underpaid their taxes and they owe money.

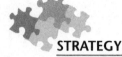

STRATEGY

Search for information that reveals the purpose of the correspondence.

THINK

- The document lists both more taxes owed than payments and credits. This means that (D) is the correct response. (C) correctly identifies that the taxpayers owe the government, but it attributes the debt to overpayment, not underpayment.

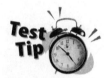

Test Tip

Note that (A) and (B) can be ruled out as answer choices because they both specify a refund rather than an amount owed.

2.2

Problem 3:

What can you infer about the marriage status of the taxpayers?

A) They are unmarried because they have different last names.

B) They are unmarried because they have different social security numbers.

C) They are married because they are filing jointly.

D) They are married but are filing separately.

STRATEGY

Use common sense and the information on the form to draw conclusions.

THINK

- (A) and (B) must be incorrect because it is common for people to be married but have different last names.

- It seems clear that the individuals are married, but are they filing jointly or separately? The IRS is addressing them together and sending them a bill together. If they were filing separately, each person would have a different tax status and would not be sent a joint document.

- It is clear that because the form is addressed to both individuals, the individuals are married, and the individuals are filing together (jointly) that (D) is incorrect, making (C) the correct response.

2.2

Problem 4:

Lisa has a question about this assessment and calls the IRS. The person she is talking to cannot find her file using her social security number or her husband's social security number. What should Lisa do?

A) Provide the record locator: PL142578194004.

B) Provide her email address.

C) Provide her home address and phone number.

D) Provide the last four digits of the record locator: 4004.

STRATEGY

Look for an item in the document that will identify Lisa and Ralph.

THINK

- Tax records typically do not use an email address (B) or a home address and phone number (C) to identify taxpayers.

- The record locator can be used to track down this document. It poses no security risk to Lisa or Ralph, so Lisa can provide the entire number rather than just the last four digits (D), making (A) the correct response.

C. Printed Documents: Labels: Problems

The following questions refer to the image shown. They pertain to reading an **ingredients label** for breakfast cereal.

Nutrition Facts

Serving Size (343g)
Servings Per Container

Amount Per Serving

Calories 310   Calories from Fat 60

	% Daily Value*
Total Fat 6g	**9%**
Saturated Fat 1g	**5%**
Trans Fat 0g	
Cholesterol 0mg	**0%**
Sodium 70mg	**3%**
Total Carbohydrate 58g	**19%**
Dietary Fiber 7g	**28%**
Sugars 23g	
Protein 5g	

Vitamin A 15%   •   Vitamin C 6%

Calcium 30%   •   Iron 15%

*Percent Daily Values are based on a 2,000 calorie diet. Your daily values may be higher or lower depending on your calorie needs:

	Calories:	2,000	2,500
Total Fat	Less than	65g	80g
Saturated Fat	Less than	20g	25g
Cholesterol	Less than	300mg	300mg
Sodium	Less than	2,400mg	2,400mg
Total Carbohydrate		300g	375g
Dietary Fiber		25g	30g

Calories per gram:
Fat 9   •   Carbohydrate 4   •   Protein 4

2.2

Problem 5:

The doctor has requested that an underweight patient have a high-calorie, low-fat diet. Is this cereal appropriate if it accounts for one-third of his diet?

A) No because the cereal is too high in both calories and fat.

B) No because the cereal is appropriately low in fat but not high enough in calories.

C) Yes because the cereal is appropriately low in fat and appropriately high in calories.

D) Yes because the cereal is appropriately high in fat and appropriately low in calories.

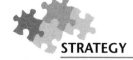

STRATEGY

Go over the entire label looking for clues about the appropriate number of calories and fat that the patient should receive.

THINK

- The label states that the cereal provides 9% of a person's daily recommended fat intake or 6 g of a standard 65 g total for fat. If the cereal represents one-third of the patient's diet, the fat intake from this cereal is low. So with regard to fat, the cereal is appropriate.

- With regard to calories, the cereal provides only 310 calories, far less than the 2500-calorie diet printed near the bottom of the label. This means with regard to calories, the cereal is too low and not appropriate.

- Being appropriate for fat but too low for calories matches answer choice (B).

2.2

Problem 6:

The patient has diabetes, and his doctor recommends that he eat fewer than 200 g of carbohydrate each day. Is this cereal a good choice for the patient who eats three meals a day?

A) Yes because the 58 g of carbohydrate represents less than one third of a 200-g total.

B) Yes because the 58 g of carbohydrate represents less than the 200-g total for the day.

C) No because the 58 g of carbohydrate represents more than one third of a 200-g total.

D) No because the 58 g of carbohydrate represents far too few carbohydrates per day for a person with diabetes.

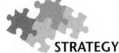

STRATEGY

Because this patient has diabetes, ignore the 300-g recommendation for carbohydrates on the label when evaluating the situation.

THINK

- Assume that the cereal represents one third of the patient's diet. Multiply the carbohydrate count by 3. If the total exceeds 200 g, then the cereal is not a good choice. If the total is less than 200 g, then the cereal is a good choice.

- 3 × 58 is equal to 171 g of carbohydrate, well under the limit of 200 g for people with diabetes, so this cereal is a good choice, making answer choice (A) correct. (B) is incorrect because it compares the 58 g with the entire day's 200-g total. (C) and (D) are incorrect because they judge the cereal not to be appropriate.

2.2

Problem 7:

How many calories from protein does a person who eats this cereal obtain?

A) 20   B) 68   C) 252   D) 0

STRATEGY

Find the number of grams of proteins that the cereal provides. Then use the number of calories per gram of protein to compute calories from protein.

THINK

- The middle section of the label shows that the cereal provides 5 g of protein.
- The bottom section of the label shows that the protein provides 4 calories per gram.
- Multiply 5 g of protein by 4 calories per gram to get 20 calories from protein, making (A) the correct response.

2.2

Problem 8:

If this cereal is served to this patient with skim milk, which totals will stay the same?

A) Fat   B) Calories   C) Carbohydrates   D) Protein

STRATEGY

Use your knowledge of the nutritional value of skim milk to find the answer.

THINK

- Skim milk has normal milk proteins and carbohydrates but no fat. Therefore, you would expect the number of calories (B), carbohydrates (C), and protein (D) to go up when the cereal is served with milk. However, the fat total when served with milk should not change, making (A) the correct answer choice.

2.2

Problem 9:

Which writing type does this label qualify as?

A) Narrative   B) Expository   C) Technical   D) Persuasive

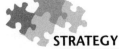

STRATEGY

Go to section 2.1 F, Types of Text, and review the categories. Find the category that fits best.

Texts generally have one of four basic forms: a **narrative** tells a story or relates a sequence of events, an **expository** piece explains or describes something, **technical** writing provides highly detailed information on a topic, and **persuasive** writing attempts to build a case for a point of view and sway the views of the reader.

THINK

- A narrative (A) tells a story, and this label clearly does not tell a story. This label contains information, but it lacks any kind of explanation, so it does not qualify as expository writing (B). There is no element of persuasion on this label, so (D) is not correct. The label does contain a great deal of detailed technical information, so it best fits a technical writing model (C).

2.3 DIRECTIONS

A. Following Directions: Overview

1. **Read:** The first thing to do is read the directions carefully without attempting to carry out any of the instructions.

2. **Step by step:** After you understand the general thrust of the directions, go step by step through each instruction.

3. **Write:** As you carry out the instructions, mark each step. Write notes, circle, or underline as necessary. If you need to make calculations, make sure you put them on paper.

4. **Diagram:** In many cases, drawing a diagram will help you understand and carry out the instructions.

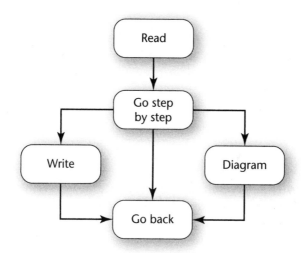

5. **Go back:** When you have finished, go back over the directions to make sure that you have followed them correctly and reached a goal that makes sense.

B. Following Directions: Problems

2.3

Problem 1:

Follow the directions.

1. Start with the words USERS KID.

2. Reverse the order of the words.

3. Insert the letter N *after* the first vowel in the first word and *before* the first vowel in the second word.

4. Place the fifth letter in the second word after the first vowel in that word.

Which words have you formed?

A) KIN RUSES   B) DINK NURSES

C) INK RUSES   D) KIND NURSES

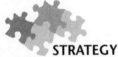

STRATEGY

Follow the steps in the Overview above. Writing as you go through the steps should be helpful for this problem.

THINK

- Write the words: USERS KID.

- Reverse the word order: KID USERS.

- Insert N in two places: KI**N**D **N**USERS

- Move the fifth letter, R, to follow the first vowel, U, in the second word: KIND NU**R**SES.

- Write out the words: KIND NURSES, making (D) the correct answer choice.

2.3

Problem 2:

Follow the directions.

1. Imagine a 4 × 4 grid made of 16 squares.

2. Remove any one of the inner squares and place it below the square on the left corner of the grid.

3. Remove any one of the inner squares and place it below the square you just repositioned.

4. Repeat step 3 with two additional squares. Place them below the squares you repositioned earlier.

Which letter have you created?

A) b   B) P   C) q   D) G

STRATEGY

Draw a diagram to visualize the steps.

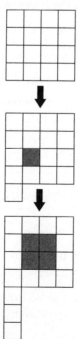

THINK

- As in step 2, move one square and place it below the square on the left corner of the grid.

- Continue the pattern with three additional squares. As you can see, a "P" is created, meaning that answer choice (B) is the correct response.

2.3

Problem 3:

Follow the directions.

1. A nurse begins with a container that has 50 ml of water.

2. The nurse adds 10 ml of medication to the container to make a solution.

3. The nurse empties the container, pouring equal amounts the solution into a red beaker and a blue beaker.

4. The nurse pours 5 ml of the solution from the red beaker to the blue beaker.

Which statement is true?

A) Both beakers have an equal volume of solution.

B) The blue beaker has more solution than the red beaker.

C) The red beaker has more solution than the blue beaker.

D) The red beaker has twice as much solution as the blue beaker.

STRATEGY

Go through the steps carefully. Draw a diagram to visualize the steps.

THINK

- After step 2, what is the volume of the container? You have added 10 ml to 50 ml to make 60 ml.

- After step 3, what is the volume of each beaker? You split 60 ml equally into two beakers, so each has 30 ml.

- After step 4, what is the volume of each beaker? You have subtracted 5 ml from the 30 ml in the red beaker and added 5 ml to the 30 ml in the blue beaker. This leaves the red beaker with 25 ml and the blue beaker with 35 ml.

- From above, it should be clear that the blue beaker has a greater volume than the red beaker, meaning that answer choice (B) is correct.

2.4 COMPARISON

A. Overview

1. **Assess:** Make an overall assessment. Look for differences and similarities between categories. For example, in comparing bicycles, one bike might have 8 gears, and another might have 12.

2. **Assign values:** Evaluate the differences between categories. For example, does having 12 gears make one bike more valuable than another? If possible, give numeric weights to your evaluations.

3. **Compare category by category:** Again, look for differences and similarities and evaluate them. Make calculations, if appropriate.

4. **Make a final judgment:** Based on the differences between items and the values you assigned, make a judgment. If appropriate, base your final judgment on the calculations you made.

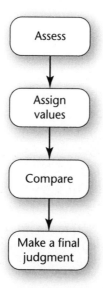

B. Problems

Use the pay scale shown here for the next four problems.

A job offers two different pay scales. Workers can choose a straight hourly pay of $25 per hour for an 8-hour day, with no extra compensation for overtime. Alternatively, workers can choose a $20 per hour basic scale but receive time and a half for overtime hours.

Scale	Hourly Pay	Overtime Pay
1	$25	$25
2	$20	Double time
3	$15	Triple time

2.4

Problem 1:

Connie is considering scale 1 or scale 2. Which scale should she choose for a 10-hour shift?

A) Scale 1 pays $10 more than scale 2.

B) Scale 1 and scale 2 pay the same.

C) Scale 2 pays $20 more than scale 1.

D) Scale 1 pays $30 more than scale 2.

STRATEGY

Compute the pay for 10 hours and compare.

THINK

- Find 10-hour pay for scale 1 and scale 2.
- For 10 hours, scale 1 pays 10 × $25 = $250, and scale 2 pays (8 × $20) + (2 × $40) = $160 + $80 = $240.
- So scale 1 pays $10 more, making it the best choice and making (A) the correct response.

2.4

Problem 2:

For a 12-hour shift which scale should Connie choose?

A) Scale 1   B) Scale 2

C) Scale 3   D) All three scales pay the same amount.

STRATEGY

Compute the pay for 12 hours and compare.

THINK

- Find 12-hour pay for scale 1, scale 2, and scale 3.

- For 12 hours, scale 1 pays 12 × $25 = $300.

- Scale 2 pays (8 × $20) + (4 × $40) = $160 + $160 = $320.

- Scale 3 pays (8 × $15) + (4 × $45) = $120 + $180 = $300

- So scale 2 pays $20 more than both scale 1 and scale 3, making (B) the correct response.

2.4

Problem 3:

When would it first pay off for Connie to choose scale 3?

A) After 10 hours   B) After 12 hours

C) After 16 hours   D) After 24 hours

STRATEGY

Make a table and compare pay.

THINK

- Construct a table like the one shown.

Scale	10 hr	11 hr	12 hr	14 hr	16 hr	17 hr
1	$250	$275	$300	$350	$400	$425
2	$240	$280	$320	$400	$480	$520
3	$210	$255	$300	$390	$480	$525

- You can see that scale 3 is gradually catching up with the other two scales as time increases.

- Scale 3 finally matches scale 1 after 12 hours and scale 2 after 16 hours.

- Beyond 16 hours, scale 3 pays more than scale 1 or 2, making (C) the correct response.

2.4

Problem 4:

What is the most Connie can earn if she works a full 24-hour shift?

A) $600   B) $800   C) $840   D) $1040

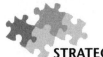

STRATEGY

Compute pay for a full 24-hour shift.

THINK

- For 24 hours, scale 1 pays 24 × $25 = $600.

- Scale 2 pays (8 × $20) + (16 × $40) = $160 + $640 = $800.

- Scale 3 pays (8 × $15) + (16 × $45) = $120 + $720 = $840

- So scale 3 pays most, making (C) the correct response.

2.5 GRAPHIC REPRESENTATIONS

A. Overview

1. **Identify:** There are many different ways to present information graphically. The most common forms include graphs, charts, tables, maps, and instrument scales.

2. **Visualize:** Before analyzing the graphic in any detail, get a "big picture" assessment of its overall meaning. If the graphic is a line graph, is it trending up or down? If the graphic is an instrument scale, what are the units it is measuring? If it is a map, what is it depicting, and what is the map scale?

3. **Problem:** On the TEAS, graphics always are accompanied by a problem. Identify the problem you are you being asked to solve. Ask yourself, how can I use the graphic to solve the problem?

4. **Trends:** In a Reading Comprehension section, you will not be asked to make complicated analyses or calculations. Instead, you will be asked about general trends and how they relate to the problem you have been asked to solve.

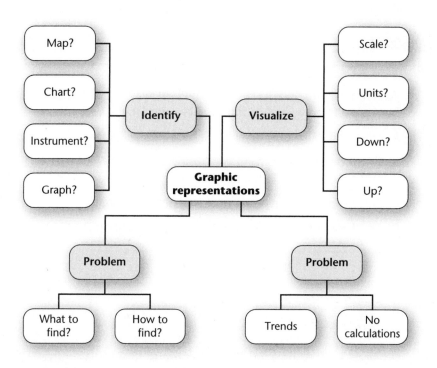

B. Maps: Problems

Use the map to answer the following questions. Assume that you are located at position "A" on Piermont Drive.

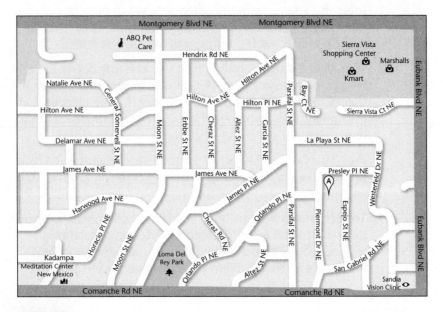

2.5

Problem 1:

Which of the following identifies the best way to get to Eubank Boulevard from your location on Piermont Drive?

A) North on Piermont, right on San Gabriel to Eubank

B) South on Piermont, right on Presley, right on Westerfeld, left on San Gabriel to Eubank

C) South on Piermont, west on Comanche to Eubank

D) South on Piermont, left on San Gabriel to Eubank

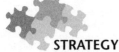

STRATEGY

Follow each route. Find the simplest and best route.

THINK

- Answer choice (A) is incorrect because going north on Piermont will not take you to San Gabriel.

- Answer choice (B) is incorrect because going south on Piermont will not take you to Presley.

- Answer choice (C) is incorrect because going west on Comanche will take you away from Eubank, not toward Eubank.

- Answer choice (D) is correct because it takes you to the intersection of San Gabriel and Eubank.

2.5

Problem 2:

Suppose you want to get to Montgomery Boulevard but you can't travel on Hendrix Road or across Hendrix Road because the entire road is blocked off because of a water main break. How would you head out to reach Montgomery?

A) From Piermont, head south to Comanche.

B) From Piermont, head west on Orlando and then make a right on Harwood.

C) Head north on Piermont and then make a right on Presley.

D) From Piermont, head west on Orlando and then north on Parsifal.

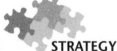

STRATEGY

Follow each route. Find the simplest and best route.

THINK

- Answer choices (B), (C), and (D) all will eventually either be on Hendrix or need to cross Hendrix in order to get to Montgomery.

- That leaves (A) as the only correct response. You would take Comanche east to Eubank and then go north on Eubank until you hit Montgomery.

C. Weight Scales: Problems

Use the scale to answer the following questions.

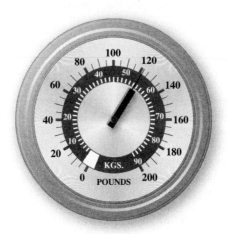

2.5

Problem 3:

Approximately how much does this patient weigh?

A) 50 kg   B) 121 lb   C) 122 lb   D) 54 kg

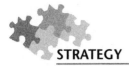

STRATEGY

Find the answer choice that matches the scale.

THINK

- The needle is pointing exactly on 55 kg, but 55 kg is not one of the answer choices.

- The needle is pointing to just over 121 lb. It is closer to 121 lb than to 122 lb, so 121 is the best estimate, making answer choice (B) the correct response.

2.5

Problem 4:

Using this same scale, a nurse weighs a man and comes up with a weight of about 70 kg. Which of the following is the best estimate for the man's weight in pounds?

A) 150 lb   B) 80 lb   C) 120 lb   D) 200 lb

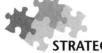

STRATEGY

Use the standard conversion between kilograms and pounds to make a very rough estimate. You don't need to make any calculations.

THINK

- 1 kg = 2.2 lb. Therefore, if the man weighs just over 70 kg, he should weigh somewhat more than twice 70 in pounds.

- 2 × 70 = 140. The man should weigh somewhat over 140 lb. 150 lb is a good estimate, so (A) is the correct answer choice.

D. Graphs: Problems

Use the graph to answer the following questions.

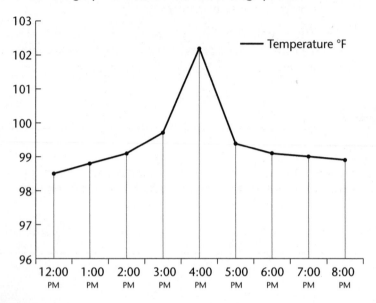

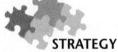

Problem 5:

At what time did the patient's temperature spike?

A) After 2 PM   B) After 3 PM   C) After 4 PM   D) Before 5 PM

STRATEGY

Read the graph and interpret the data.

THINK

- The temperature spike should be interpreted when the graph rose most steeply.

- The steepest rise on the graph occurs just after 3 PM. This makes answer choice (B) the correct response.

2.5

Problem 6:

A nurse administered acetaminophen at 3:20 PM. For how long did the patient's temperature continue to rise?

A) About 1 hour   B) About 20 minutes

C) About 1.5 hours   D) About 40 minutes

STRATEGY

Read the graph and interpret the data.

THINK

- The 3:20 time period is about one third of the way between 3 and 4 PM.

- The patient's temperature reached a maximum at 4 PM. This was about 40 minutes after the acetaminophen was given. That makes answer choice (D) the correct response.

2.5

Problem 7:

What was the difference between the patient's maximum temperature and the minimum temperature after the acetaminophen was given?

A) 3.2°F   B) 2.2°F   C) 5.0°F   D) 1.5°F

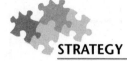

STRATEGY

Read the graph and interpret the data.

THINK

- The maximum temperature at 4 PM was about 102.1°F. The minimum temperature afterward at 8 PM was about 98.9°F.

- Subtracting: 102.1 − 98.9 = 3.2°F. That makes answer choice (A) the correct response.

English and Language Usage

PARTS OF SPEECH

A. Nouns and Verbs

1. A **noun** is a word for a person, place, or thing. The nouns in this sentence are underlined.

    My <u>brother</u> <u>Frank</u> bought two <u>fishing poles</u> and a <u>bucket</u> of <u>worms</u>.

2. A **proper noun** is the official name of a person, place, or thing. Proper nouns are always capitalized. Examples of proper nouns include *Frank, Iowa, Vice President,* and *Yankee Stadium.*

3. Compound nouns include two or more words. Examples: *fishing poles, maple tree,* and *Hartley Park*

4. Plural nouns identify more than one item. Note that some plural nouns do not end in the letter *s.* Examples: *fishing poles, worms, children,* and *people*

5. A **verb** is a word that shows action or a state of being. The verbs in this sentence are underlined.

    The dog <u>barked</u> and <u>howled</u>, but Hannah <u>was</u> so tired that she <u>did</u> not <u>wake</u> up.

6. Action verbs show action. Action verbs in the sentence above are *barked, howled,* and *wake.*

7. Verbs of being (linking verbs) include forms of *to be, to seem, to appear,* and a few others. In the sentence above, the word *was* is a verb of being.

8. Helping verbs do not stand by themselves. Helping verbs are parts of other verbs. Examples: *<u>is</u> eating, <u>have</u> finished, <u>did</u> not wake, <u>can</u> win, <u>should</u> know.* In the sentence above, *did* is a helping verb that helps *wake.*

9. Verbs take on a different tense depending on the situation.

	Present	Past	Future
Simple	I talk.	I talked.	I will talk.
Perfect	I have talked.	I had talked.	I will have talked.
Continuous	I am talking.	I was talking.	I will be talking.
Continuous perfect	I have been talking.	I had been talking.	I will have been talking.

10. The **past participle** is the verb form that is used with helping verbs *have* such as *have <u>worked</u>* or *has <u>brought</u>*. The **present participle** shows ongoing action with *is* such as *was <u>hoping</u>* or *is <u>sleeping</u>*.

11. Irregular verbs have unusual forms. Here are a few of them.

		Participle				Participle	
Present	Past	Past	Present	Present	Past	Past	Present
eat	ate	eaten	eating	blow	blew	blown	blowing
speak	spoke	spoken	speaking	bring	brought	brought	bringing
sing	sang	sung	singing	put	put	put	putting
do	did	done	doing	hide	hid	hidden	hiding
see	saw	seen	seeing	show	showed	shown	showing
lie	lay	lain	lying	lay	laid	laid	laying
keep	kept	kept	keeping	grow	grew	grown	growing

3.1

Problem 1:

How is the word *lights* being used in the following sentence?

The <u>lights</u> go out, and the room stays dark until Jeremy <u>lights</u> a candle.

A) First as a verb; then as a noun

B) First as a noun; then as a verb

C) As a noun both times

D) As a verb both times

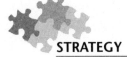

STRATEGY

Refer to the definitions of nouns and verbs.

THINK

- When the lights go out, *lights* is referring to a thing, so it is being used as a noun. When Jeremy *lights,* he is performing an action, so *lights* is being used as a verb.

- This makes (B) the correct answer choice.

3.1

Problem 2:

Which sentence is correct?

A) He has brung refreshments to the party that I have seen.

B) I seen him bring refreshments to the party.

C) He has brought refreshments to the party that I seen.

D) I have seen him bring refreshments to the party.

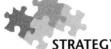

STRATEGY

Refer to the irregular verb forms.

THINK

- In (A), the sentence uses *brung,* an incorrect verb form, so it is incorrect.

- Both (B) and (C) use the word *seen* as a past tense verb rather than a past participle, so they are incorrect.

- Answer choice (D) uses the past participle form of *seen* correctly and the present form of *bring,* so it is correct.

B. Pronouns

1. A **pronoun** is a word that takes the place of a noun. **Personal pronouns** refer to specific person.

   <u>Maude</u> read the newspaper before <u>she</u> ate breakfast.

2. The pronoun *she* above refers to Maude. The person that a personal pronoun refers to is called the **antecedent**.

3. **Possessive pronouns** show ownership.

   That pizza you ate was <u>mine</u>.

   The best plan was <u>his</u>, but the most creative plan was <u>hers</u>.

4. Pronouns and antecedents should always agree.

5. Forms of pronouns are shown in the table.

	Personal		Possessive	
	Singular	**Plural**	**Singular**	**Plural**
First person	I, me	we, us	mine	ours
Second person	you	you	yours	yours
Third person	he, she, him, her, it	they, them	his, hers, its	theirs

6. Subjective pronouns serve as **subjects (see section 3.2 A)** of sentences. Objective pronouns serve as **objects (see also section 3.1 D).**

7. The subject is the item that the phrase or sentence is about. The subject typically initiates the action. The object is the item on which the action is being initiated.

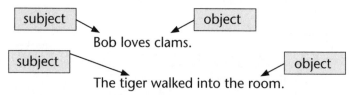

8. Subjective personal pronouns function as subjects. Objective personal pronouns function as objects.

   Subjective personal pronouns: *I, you, he, she, we, they*

   Objective personal pronouns: *me, you, him, us, her, them*

9. Pronouns and antecedents should always agree.

Examples:

<u>Him</u> and Laurie both graduated the same year.
(Incorrect—*Him*, an objective pronoun, is incorrectly being used as a subjective pronoun.)

<u>He</u> and Laurie both graduated the same year.
(Correct—*He*, a subjective pronoun, is correctly being used as a subject.)

The doctor gave a compliment to Meryl and I.
(Incorrect—*I*, a subjective pronoun, is incorrectly being used as an objective pronoun.)

The doctor gave a compliment to Meryl and me.
(Correct—*me*, an objective pronoun, is correctly being used as an object.)

3.1

Problem 3:

Which sentence best fixes the sentence below?

The coach warned each player to have fun before they entered the game.

A) The coach warned each player to have fun before he or she entered the game.

B) The coach warned each player to have fun before she entered the game.

C) The coach warned each player to have fun before he entered the game.

D) The sentence is correct.

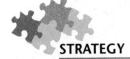

STRATEGY

Make sure that the pronoun agrees with its antecedent.

THINK

- The pronoun, *they,* is plural. The antecedent, *player,* is singular. So the pronoun and antecedent do not agree. This means that (D) cannot be the correct answer.

- To fix the sentence, you can make the pronoun singular. Choices (B) and (C) are grammatically correct, but there is no way of knowing whether the players were male or female. So neither choice is best.

- Answer choice (A) is grammatically correct, and it does not erroneously assign gender to the player, so it is the correct choice.

- **Test tips:** Pay close attention to when a question asks for "best" answer. It often means that some answer choices might be acceptable but that other choices are clearly superior.

3.1

Problem 4:

Which sentence is correct?

A) Both Eric and me ask that you give him and me a break.

B) Both Eric and I ask that you give him and me a break.

C) Both Eric and I ask that you give him and I a break.

D) Both Eric and me ask that you give he and I a break.

STRATEGY

Make sure that the correct subjective and objective pronouns are used.

THINK

- The subjective *Eric* and *I* must be used as the subject of the sentence, not the objective *Eric* and *me,* so both (A) and (D) are incorrect.

- *Him* and *me* are objects in this case—they are receiving the break—so the objective form should be used. This makes (B) the correct response and eliminates (C) because it uses the subjective *I* in an objective situation.

C. Adjectives and Adverbs

1. An **adjective** is a word that modifies a noun or a pronoun.

    I left the <u>red</u> scissors in the <u>middle</u> drawer on the <u>right</u> side of the refrigerator.

2. In the sentence above, *red* modifies *scissors, middle* modifies *drawer,* and *right* modifies *side.*

3. An **adverb** modifies a verb, adjective, or another adverb.

    Walter <u>very</u> <u>carefully</u> lifted the lid off the <u>bright</u> yellow coffee cup and saw that it was empty.

4. In the sentence above, *carefully* modifies the verb *lifted, bright* modifies the adjective *yellow,* and *very* modifies the adverb *carefully.*

5. Adverbs often tell *when, how, where,* or *how much.*

    Jill awakens by 5 AM, runs <u>down</u> to the river, and <u>then</u> returns <u>before</u> she eats breakfast.

    In the sentence above, the adverbs *down, then,* and *before* tell you where and when events occur.

3.1

Problem 5:

Which statement is true of the following sentence?

Quite often Paula speaks hastily and makes an extremely big mistake.

A) Adjective *often* modifies adjective *hastily.*

B) Adverb *quite* modifies verb *speaks.*

C) Adverb *extremely* modifies adjective *big.*

D) Adverb *extremely* modifies verb *speaks.*

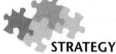

STRATEGY

Refer to the definitions of both adjectives and adverbs.

THINK

- Answer choice (A) can be eliminated because *often* is not an adjective.

- *Quite* modifies *often,* not the verb *speaks,* so (B) is incorrect.

- The adverb *extremely* modifies the adjective *big,* not the verb *speaks,* so (D) is incorrect, and (C) is the correct answer choice.

D. Prepositions

1. **Prepositions** are the small words such as *for, in, at, from, of, out, before*, after, since,* and *with* that define relationships between other words and phrases in a sentence.

2. Prepositions are always followed by an **object**, a noun or noun phrase that is the object of the preposition.

3. The prepositions below are underlined. The objects of the prepositions are double underlined.

   Steve walked <u>into</u> the <u>barn</u>.

   <u>After</u> the <u>storm</u>, Nita fell asleep.

   Congress focused <u>on getting</u> things done.

   > The word *getting* functions as a noun here.

4. Some words can function as both prepositions and adverbs. If the word has an object, it is a preposition. If the word does not have an object, it is an adverb.

   Dave looked <u>down</u>. (Adverb: no object)

   Dave looked <u>down</u> the hall. (Preposition with object: the hall)

5. Objects of prepositions always take the objective case.

   Marnie gave the money to <u>he</u>.
   (Incorrect—subjective pronoun *he*.)

   Marnie gave the money to <u>him</u>.
   (Correct—objective pronoun *him*.)

---

*Some words, such as *before* and *after*, can be used as both prepositions and adverbs.

3.1

Problem 6:

Which statement is true of this sentence?

Paul looked up and saw that Keesha had dropped her paddle into the water.

A) *Up* is used as a preposition, and *into* is used as an adverb.

B) Both *up* and *into* are used as prepositions.

C) *Up* is used as an adverb, and *into* is used as a preposition.

D) Both *up* and *into* are used as adverbs..

STRATEGY

Refer to the distinction between adverbs and prepositions.

THINK

- *Up* is clearly an adverb because it has no object. This rules out both (A) and (B).

- *Into* clearly has an object—the word *water*. So (D) cannot be correct. This leaves (C) as the correct response.

3.1

Problem 7:

Which sentence is correct?

A) The performance was intended exclusively for Warren and I.

B) The performance was exclusively intended for Warren and I.

C) The performance was intended exclusively for me and he.

D) The performance was intended exclusively for Warren and me.

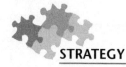

STRATEGY

Refer to the rule that objects of prepositions must take the objective case.

THINK

- Answer choices (A) and (B) are incorrect because the object of the preposition, *for,* is a subjective pronoun, *I,* instead of an objective pronoun.

- Choice (C) includes one objective pronoun, *me,* but also uses a subjective pronoun, *he,* so it is incorrect.

- Choice (D) is correct because it uses the objective *me* as the object of the preposition.

3.2 SENTENCES

A. Subjects and Predicates

1. A **sentence** uses a subject and a predicate to express a complete thought.

   Anna and her company issued dividends to all stockholders.

2. The **subject** of the sentence above identifies whom or what the sentence is about. The subject of the sentence above is underlined.

3. The **predicate** is the phrase that identifies action in a sentence. The predicate always includes the verb of the sentence. In the sentence below, the predicate is underlined.

   Unlike his brother, Patrick enjoyed practicing the piano.

4. The subject of the sentence must always identify what the sentence is actually about. The predicate must always identify the action of the subject.

   When the rain became heavy, Marly opened her umbrella.

5. The subject above is Marly, not the rain. So the predicate goes with the subject: *opened her umbrella.*

3.2

Problem 1:

What is the predicate of the following sentence?

When the curtain went down, the audience exploded into a chorus of boos and jeers.

A) exploded

B) went down

C) exploded into a chorus of boos and jeers

D) exploded into a chorus

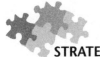

STRATEGY

Refer to the definition of a predicate.

THINK

- A predicate includes the verb and the phrase that goes with the verb.

- The predicate must identify the action that the subject of the sentence is taking. The subject of this sentence is the audience, not the curtain, so although *went down* is a verb phrase ,it does not identify the action of the sentence, making (B) incorrect.

- Choices (A) and (D) identify part of the predicate but not the entire phrase, so they are incorrect. (C) includes the entire action phrase, so it is the correct answer choice.

B. Types of Sentence and Voice

1. A **declarative** sentence makes a statement and ends with a period.

   The moon makes a journey across the sky every night.

   Photographers call the late afternoon light the "golden light."

2. An **interrogative** sentence asks a question and ends with a question mark.

   Are you going to finish the job by Friday?

   How many young men and women today are interested in joining the military?

3. An **exclamatory** sentence expresses excitement or strong feelings and ends with an exclamation point.

   Look how much things have changed!

   The Dallas Cowboys are the champions!

4. A **command** gives an order, makes a request, or gives instructions. Commands can end with periods or exclamation points. Commands often have an implied subject of "you" that is not explicitly stated.

   Before <u>you</u> lock up, check every window and door and then set the alarm. (Stated subject: *you*)

   Go one block past Webster Avenue, turn right, and then look for a white stucco house. (Unstated subject: *you*)

5. Sentences have a point of view or voice.

   I never forgot who helped me on my first day at the hospital. (**First-person voice:** "I" and "me" voice)

   You gain confidence and you start thinking that you can accomplish things that others can't. (**Second-person voice:** "You" voice)

   McClintock first became interested in genetics in high school. (**Third-person voice:** "He," "she," "they" voice)

6. The voice in a sentence can be passive or active. In the active voice, the subject is clearly identified, and active, direct verbs are used.

   Monica checked the monitor, adjusted the IV drip, plumped up the patient's pillows, and smiled. (**Active voice:** *Monica* is clearly initiating the action of checking, adjusting, plumping, and smiling.)

7. In the passive voice, the initiator of the action is not clearly identified. Passive verbs with *is* or *was* are used (*is* done, *was* given, *were* felt).

> The monitor was checked, the IV drip was adjusted, and the patient's pillows were plumped. (**Passive voice:** No one is identified as the person checking, adjusting, or plumping.)

3.2

Problem 2:

Which description best characterizes the following sentence?

Mistakes were clearly made and excuses were provided, but nothing was done to improve patient care at this hospital.

A) Interrogative sentence, passive, first-person voice

B) Declarative sentence, active, second-person voice

C) Declarative sentence, passive, third-person voice

D) Command, passive, third-person voice

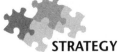

STRATEGY

Refer to the different types of sentence and voice.

THINK

- The sentence clearly is a statement rather than a question or a command, so (A) and (D) can be eliminated.

- The voice is clearly passive because it features passive verbs—*were made, were provided, was done*. The voice is also clearly not first person because the narrator is un-named and there is no *I* or *me* element. This means that (B) is incorrect, and (C) is the correct answer choice.

C. Clauses and Phrases

1. Sentences can include clauses and phrases. **Clauses** have both a subject (noun) and a verb, but **phrases** may have one lack one or both of these items.

2. A clause is underlined below, and a phrase is double underlined.

   When Bethany grabbed the steering wheel, the boat began to veer wildly in every direction.

3. **Independent clauses** can stand on their own as complete sentences. A **simple sentence** consists of a single independent clause.

4. A complex sentence has more than one clause. Clauses are often introduced by a coordinating conjunction. **Coordinating conjunctions** include *and, so, but, for, or, nor,* and *yet.*

   The dog started to panic after the fireworks started, so we had to leave early.

5. Both clauses above are independent. They are separated by the coordinating conjunction *so.* The main clause is *we had to leave early.*

6. Connecting words (e.g., conjunctive adverbs) such as *also, however, furthermore, nevertheless, consequently,* and *therefore* can also introduce independent clauses.

   The budget crisis was averted; however, a new showdown on the deficit loomed only a few months in the future.

7. **Dependent clauses** (subordinate) have a subject and a verb but make no sense on their own without the rest of the sentence.

   As Rome was burning, Nero supposedly played his fiddle.

8. The underlined clause above has a subject and verb but makes no sense on its own: *As Rome was burning.* So it is a dependent clause.

9. Dependent clauses can be used as nouns, adjectives, and adverbs.

> Mike, <u>the bass player who is from Tennessee</u>, loves country music. (Adjectival clause modifies *Mike*.)

> The cat leaves a strong odor <u>wherever she goes</u>. (Adverbial clause modifies *leaves*.)

> <u>Whatever you're looking for</u> is not in this document. (Noun clause functions as subject of the sentence.)

3.2

Problem 3:

Which of the following is true of this sentence?

Although Senator Simpson is now obsessed with budgetary deficits, when he was in power, he saw nothing wrong with running a deficit.

A) *Senator Simpson is now obsessed with budgetary deficits* is an independent clause.

B) *Although Senator Simpson is now obsessed with budgetary deficits* is a dependent clause.

C) *When he was in power* is an independent clause.

D) *He saw nothing wrong with running a deficit* is a dependent clause.

STRATEGY

Refer to the definitions of both dependent and independent clauses.

THINK

- An independent clause must be able to stand on its own as a sentence. *Although Senator Simpson is now obsessed with budgetary deficits* and *when he was in power* cannot stand on their own, so neither clause is independent, making (A) and (C) incorrect.

- *He saw nothing wrong with running a deficit* can stand on its own, so it is independent, not dependent, making (D) incorrect.

- As stated above, *Although Senator Simpson is now obsessed with budgetary deficits* and *when he was in power* cannot stand on its own, so (B) correctly identifies it as a dependent clause.

D. Sentence Errors

1. **Run-on sentences** and **comma splice** sentences contain two independent clauses that are not connected and not separated by appropriate punctuation.

   The phone is very well engineered it lacks adequate software. (Incorrect: run-on)

   The phone is very well engineered, it lacks adequate software. (Incorrect: comma splice)

   The phone is very well engineered. However, it lacks adequate software. (Correct)

   The phone is very well engineered, but it lacks adequate software. (Correct)

   Although the phone is very well engineered, it lacks adequate software. (Correct)

   The phone is very well engineered; however, it lacks adequate software. (Correct)

2. **Sentence fragments** are "sentences" that contain incomplete thoughts, often because a dependent clause is expressed as a sentence.

   He can juggle four balls. <u>While riding a unicycle</u>. (Fragment)

   He can juggle four balls while riding a unicycle. (Correct)

   <u>Because it rained for seven hours</u>. The basement flooded. (Fragment)

   The basement flooded because it rained for seven hours. (Correct)

3.2

Problem 4:

Which sentence is correct?

A) Although Mr. Benes was now walking normally, he was still kept in rehab.

B) Although Mr. Benes was now walking normally; he was still kept in rehab.

C) Although Mr. Benes was now walking normally. He was still kept in rehab.

D) Although Mr. Benes was now walking normally; however, he was still kept in rehab.

STRATEGY

Refer to the definitions of fragments, run-ons, and comma splices.

THINK

- Answer choices (B), (C), and (D) all treat dependent clauses as though they were independent. By itself the clause *Although Mr. Benes was now walking normally* makes no sense, so it should not be separated by punctuation.

- Answer choice (A) correctly treats *Although Mr. Benes was now walking normally as* a dependent clause and sets it off with a comma. Therefore, it is the correct answer.

E. Sentence Agreement

1. Subjects and verbs must always agree. Some subjects, such as *both, few, many,* and *several,* are always treated as plural.

    Both <u>are</u> acceptable to me.

    <u>Many</u> have flaws or defects.

2. All of these indefinite subjects take a singular verb:

> *anybody, anyone, anything, each, either, every,*
> *everybody, everything, much, neither, nobody, no one,*
> *nothing, one, other, somebody, something, someone*

Everyone has their own way of looking at things.
(Incorrect)

Everyone has his or her own way of looking at things.
(Correct)

Neither choice was acceptable. (Correct)

Each student should clean their own plate. (Incorrect)

Each student should clean his or her own plate.
(Correct)

3. Subjects that are taken as a single unit or topic take singular verbs.

Research and development is important.
(Singular: one unit)

Research and planning are increasing each year.
(Plural: two separate categories; not one unit)

Fifty dollars is more than enough. (Singular: one unit)

Sports is a tough business to get into for a broadcaster.
(Singular: Sports is a topic.)

Different sports require entirely different skill sets.
(Plural: more than one sport)

Some of the money has already been spent.
(Singular: *Some* refers to a singular amount.)

Some of my stamps are worth more than a hundred
dollars. (Plural: *Some* refers to multiple stamps.)

Half of the medical team is on call this week.
(Singular: team as a unit)

Half of the members of the medical team call in
sick on Monday. (Plural: refers to more than one
individual)

3.2

Problem 5:

Which sentence is correct?

A) Three-fourths of the staff are underpaid.

B) Three-fourths of the staff is underpaid.

C) Three-fourths of the staff members is underpaid.

D) Three-fourths of the 12-person staff are underpaid.

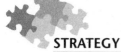 **STRATEGY**

Refer to the principles outlined above about sentence agreement.

THINK

- In (A), (D), and (B), the staff is being considered as a single unit, so the sentence should take a singular verb, making (B) the correct response.

- In (C), the staff is being considered as many individuals, so a plural verb should be used.

3.2

Problem 6:

Which sentence is correct?

A) Everybody has the right to their opinion.

B) We all has the right to do as we please.

C) Everybody has the right to his or her opinion.

D) No one have the right to be disrespectful.

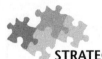

STRATEGY

Refer to the principles outlined on the previous page about sentence agreement.

THINK

- In (B) and (D), the verb form is mismatched. In (B), *We* should have a plural verb, but in (D), *No one* should take a singular verb.

- In (A) and (C), *Everybody* is singular, so *his or her* should be used rather than *their*. This makes (C) the correct response.

3.3 PUNCTUATION AND CAPITALIZATION

A. Commas and Periods

1. A **period** is used to end declarative sentences (**see section 3.2. B**). Periods are also used for many abbreviations, including Dr., etc., Ms., Hon., and U.S.

2. Periods are placed inside of quotation marks (**see 3.3 B**) and parentheses if they enclose a full sentence. If parentheses do not enclose a full sentence, the period is placed outside of the quotation marks.

   We heard no barking. (The dog was asleep.)

   The recipe called for lots of healthy ingredients (and butter and sugar).

3. **Commas** are used in a variety of situations following these general rules:

   a. **Series of three or more:** Use commas to separate items.

   The patient had no money, identification, or insurance.

   We are improving our performance with respect to response time for patients, overall hospital infection rate, and family–patient interaction satisfaction.

b. **After an introductory word group:** Use commas after phrases or clauses that come before the subject.

Without any way to get home during the storm, Luther spent the night at the hospital.

Although she was trained at elite universities, Gwen was the first one in her family to attend college.

c. **Before a coordinating conjunction** (*so, but, for, or, nor, yet;* **see section 3.2 C)**

Tupac Shakur was clearly a troubled individual, but he was also clearly a genius.

Beyoncé was worried that something would go wrong, so she lip synched her performance during the Super Bowl.

d. **To mark interruptions within a sentence:** Use two commas to set off the interruption.

The Dallas Cowboys, although widely despised, are also perhaps the most popular team in the NFL.

3.3

Problem 1:

Which sentence is punctuated correctly?

A) Dave, an insightful and talented therapist, is nevertheless prone to jumping to conclusions.

B) Dave is an insightful and talented therapist but is nevertheless prone to jumping to conclusions.

C) Although Dave, is an insightful and talented therapist, he is nevertheless prone to jumping to conclusions.

D) Dave an insightful and talented therapist is nevertheless prone to jumping to conclusions.

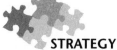

STRATEGY

Refer to the rules of punctuation cited above.

THINK

- Answer choice (B) fails to precede the coordinating conjunction *but* with a comma, so it is incorrect.

- (C) incorrectly places a comma between Dave, the subject of the sentence, and the predicate, as if the predicate were an interruption.

- (D) fails to place commas to introduce the phrase that describes Dave, so it is incorrect.

- Answer choice (A) is correct because it correctly sets off the interruption, *an insightful and talented therapist*, with commas.

B. Apostrophes and Quotation Marks

1. Use an **apostrophe** to show letters that have been left out in a contraction:

don't	you're	I'm	isn't
he's	hasn't	won't	doesn't
can't	we're	I'll	we've
you've	it's	who's	they're

2. Note these tricky examples that often cause mistakes.

	Form	Sentence
it's (contraction)	it + is	It's raining outside.
its (possessive)		My car lost its pep.
who's (contraction)	who + is	Who's hungry?
whose (interrogative)		Whose shoes are these?
you're (contraction)	you + are	You're a happy dog.
your (possessive)		This is your dog.
they're (contraction)	they + are	They're eating lunch.
their (possessive)		This is their lunch.
there (adverb)		There is your lunch.

3. Apostrophes show possession.

Hal's bicycle   Lina's job   Francis's district
Adam and Franco's Garage (belongs to both)
the members' decision (decision of more than one member)
the United States's legacy

4. Possessive pronouns don't take apostrophes.

   yours   ours   theirs   its

5. In acronyms and other unusual forms, apostrophes are used only when necessary to avoid confusion.

   1980s   PDFs   URLs
   do's and don'ts   p's and q's

6. **Quotation marks** identify a person's exact words.

7. In dialogue, a quotation is typically introduced with a comma and terminates with end punctuation. Punctuation stays inside of the end of the quotation.

   > Bonnie said, "Where have all the flowers gone?"

   > "My friend Marcus is a genius," Sally joked.

   > "Only five districts have voted!" Karl cried. "How many are left?"

8. When a quotation continues without a period, no capitalization is required.

   > "The die is cast," Churchill lamented, "and it looks like there will be war."

9. Quotation marks are also used for titles of songs, poems, and articles but not for book titles.

3.3

Problem 2:

Which item is punctuated correctly?

A) "It's clear that Michael Jordan's better than LeBron," Tanya said, "at least so far."

B) "It's clear that Michael Jordan's better than LeBron" Tanya said, "at least so far."

C) "Its clear that Michael Jordan's better than LeBron", Tanya said. "at least so far."

D) "It's clear that Michael Jordan's better than LeBron," Tanya said, "At least so far".

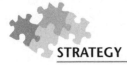

STRATEGY

Refer to the rules for apostrophes and quotations.

THINK

- You can identify (C) as incorrect because it fails to put an apostrophe in *Its*. Both (C) and (D) incorrectly place punctuation outside the end of a quotation. They also make capitalization mistakes in the word *at*, failing to capitalize in (C) and capitalizing erroneously in (D).

- (B) makes the mistake of failing to put any punctuation at the end of the first part of the quotation after *LeBron*.

- Answer choice (A) correctly applies all of the rules for apostrophes and quotations, so it is correct.

C. Colons, Semicolons, Hyphens, and Dashes

1. Use a **colon** to introduce a list, an extended quotation, an example, or a conclusion.

    > Todd instructed me to purchase these items: bread flour, yeast, cinnamon, sugar, and milk. (List)

    > John F. Kennedy famously stated: "Ask not what your country can do for you. Ask what you can do for your country." (Extended quotation)

    > The obesity data made one thing clear: Drinking soda is not good for you. (Conclusion)

    > Bonds had one big thing working against him: his rather abrasive personality. (Example)

2. Note that the first word after the colon should be capitalized only if introduces a complete sentence.

3. The **semicolon** is used to separate independent clauses that are not connected by a conjunction.

    > Jon Stewart is outrageous and sophomoric; he is also hilarious.

4. Semicolons are used with conjunctive adverbs such as *however, still, thus, nevertheless,* and *therefore* to separate independent clauses.

> A small 1 percent sliver of the population pays almost 40 percent of all federal income taxes; however, this segment owns more than 40 percent of the nation's wealth.

5. **Hyphens** are used to combine two words to create a compound modifier. The words are hyphenated only when they serve to modify a noun.

> Nora's <u>last-second</u> shot tied the score. (Hyphenated, modifies *shot*)

> Nora's big shot came at the <u>last second</u>. (Unhyphenated)

6. A **dash** is used to introduce a surprise to the end of a sentence.

> The movie featured a spectacular and subtle performance by Quvenzhané Wallis—a 5-year-old child!

7. Dashes are also used to set off an important fact or amplification of a fact.

> The legendary 396-cubic-inch Chevrolet engine—which got less than 16 miles per gallon—was symbolic of a time when gasoline was cheap and environmental concerns were nonexistent.

3.3

Problem 3:

Which sentence is punctuated correctly?

A) Rowling brought her Harry Potter manuscript to nine-different publishers and was rejected nine times, the tenth saw things differently.

B) Rowling brought her Harry Potter manuscript to nine different publishers, and was rejected, nine times: the tenth saw things differently.

C) Rowling brought her Harry-Potter manuscript to nine different publishers and was rejected nine times, the tenth: saw things differently.

D) Rowling brought her Harry Potter manuscript to nine different publishers and was rejected nine times; the tenth saw things differently.

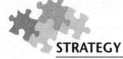

STRATEGY

Refer to the use of different kinds of punctuation outlined above.

THINK

- (A) is incorrect because it incorrectly places both a hyphen and a comma. The comma attempts to connect two independent clauses, creating what is termed a *comma splice* (**see section 3.2 D**)

- (B) incorrectly sets off a phrase, *and was rejected*, and uses a colon incorrectly.

- (C) incorrectly hyphenates *Harry Potter* and incorrectly places a colon.

- Only answer choice (D) recognizes that two independent clauses are being used here and connects them with a semicolon, so it is the correct answer choice.

D. Capitalization

1. Rules for capitalization are shown below.

Capitalize	Example
First word of a sentence or quotation	Loose lips sink ships. She sells sea shells. Tom asked, "How are you?"
Proper names and titles of individuals	Larry Dr. Juanita Grossman Mayor Michael Bloomberg Samuel Diaz, RN

(continued)

Capitalize	Example
	President Johnson "Magic" Johnson Ms. Connie West The Honorable Ethan Greenwald Uncle Marty Grandma Bessie Allah
Geographical names and ethnicities	Pittsburgh Sri Lanka Lake Erie the Upper West Side Northern Hemisphere Mount Rushmore French African American Peruvian
Calendar events and holidays	Monday Valentine's Day July Thanksgiving
Names of organizations	the United Nations the Carnegie Foundation Miami Heat Republican Party Apple Computer
Awards, ships, monuments, works of art	the Nobel Prize the Statue of Liberty Congressional Medal of Honor Golden Globe Award *U.S.S. Cole* the *Mona Lisa*
Titles (books and movies in italics; stories and songs in quotes)	*In Cold Blood* "The Lottery" "Accentuate the Positive" *The King's Speech*
Events	the Winter Olympics the French Revolution Homecoming Dance

3.3

Problem 4:

Which sentence is correct?

A) Celebrated Author Truman Capote was childhood friends in Alabama with Harper Lee, author of the pulitzer-prize-winning novel *To Kill a Mockingbird*.

B) Celebrated author Truman Capote was childhood friends in alabama with Harper Lee, author of the Pulitzer-Prize-winning novel *to kill a Mockingbird*.

C) Celebrated Author Truman Capote was childhood friends in Alabama with Harper Lee, author of the Pulitzer-Prize-Winning Novel *To Kill a Mockingbird*

D) Celebrated author Truman Capote was childhood friends in Alabama with Harper Lee, author of the Pulitzer Prize–winning novel *To Kill a Mockingbird*.

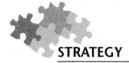

STRATEGY

Refer to the capitalization rules above.

THINK

- Both (A) and (C) make the mistake of capitalizing the word *Author*. (A) also fails to capitalize the Pulitzer Prize.

- (B) fails to capitalize the proper name of Capote's home state of Alabama and part of the title of Lee's novel, so it is incorrect.

- (D) correctly capitalizes *Alabama;* the *Pulitzer Prize;* and the name of Lee's novel, *To Kill a Mockingbird*.

SPELLING AND VOCABULARY

A. Frequently Misspelled Words

1. Words that are commonly confused with one another covered earlier (**see section 3.3**) include *its* and *it's; your* and *you're; they're, their,* and *there;* and *whose* and *who's.*

2. This table shows other words that are commonly misspelled.

Words	Common Form	Sentence
to	preposition	I am going to the store.
too	adverb	I have too many shoes.
two	number	She has two sisters.
affect	verb	Treatment affects recovery.
effect	noun	Treatment has a major effect on recovery.
accept	verb	I accept your nomination to be president.
except	preposition	We got it all done except the cleanup.
than	preposition	Mars is smaller than Earth.
then	adverb	The play began and then the lights went out.
already	adverb	I already finished my homework.
all ready	adjective	The appetizers are all ready.
stationary	adjective	The fixture was stationary.
stationery	noun	He wrote me a note on his stationery.
allusion	noun	The movie included an allusion to Tarentino.
illusion	noun	Promises of quick money often turn out to be an illusion.
principle	noun	I live by a simple principle: Be nice.
principal	noun	The principal of the school was fired.
break	verb	Two big shots break the game open.
brake	noun	I hit the brake hard on the way down the hill.

(continued)

(*continued*)

Words	Common Form	Sentence
complement	noun	Crackers are the perfect complement to soup.
compliment	verb	I compliment you on your restraint.
advise	verb	"I advise you to remain silent," the lawyer said.
advice	noun	Megan's advice was to look for a new job.
steal	verb	Employees steal pens from work frequently.
steel	noun	The bike frame was made of super-light steel.
hear	verb	You can hear the geese flying overhead.
here	adverb	The best jobs are here in Columbus.
conscious	adjective	Evan was conscious of Al's decision to quit the firm.
conscience	noun	My conscience won't let me cheat.
device	noun	The iPad was a device that few anticipated.
devise	verb	My boss can devise a plan for saving money.
eminent	adjective	Hugh Scott is an eminent scholar.
imminent	adjective	The budget showdown is imminent.

3. Other commonly misspelled words.

accommodate	aggravate	aging	aisle
allot	arctic	attendance	believe
believable	calendar	column	committee
conceivable	conscious	conscience	conscientious
coolly	curiosity	deceive	desirable
eligible	environment	exercise	exhaust
existence	fascinate	forfeit	grievous
guidance	government	incidentally	irresistible

(*continued*)

library	maintenance	marriage	miniature
muscle	necessary	obedience	occasion
occurrence	persistent	possession	preference
preference	propeller	psychiatrist	receivable
recommend	relieve	religious	repetition
representative	rechargeable	restaurant	surprise
symmetry	temperament	tendency	unnecessary

3.4

Problem 1:

Which sentence is correct?

A) Each device was rechargable accept for the toy car.

B) Each device was rechargeable except for the toy car.

C) Each devise was rechargeable except for the toy car

D) Each devise was rechargeable except for the toy car.

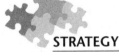

STRATEGY

Refer to the list of commonly misspelled words.

THINK

- The word *device* is being used as a noun here, so both (C) and (D) are incorrect.

- In (A), *accept* is mistakenly used as a preposition instead of *except,* so that choice is incorrect. (A) also misspells *rechargeable.*

- (B) uses *device, rechargeable,* and *except* correctly, so it is the correct response.

B. Context Clues

1. The **context clues** surrounding an unfamiliar word provide hints to the word's meaning.

2. When encountering an unfamiliar word, try these strategies to formulate a guess:

   a. Look for a **definition:**

   Carnavon then found a large jeweled cup among the treasures and assumed the goblet was the ancient king's **chalice.**

   > **chalice** = large cup, goblet

   b. Look for a **synonym:**

   > **purview** = field

   The scientist's **purview,** or primary field, was limited to molecular biology.

   c. Look for an **antonym:**

   > **chastise** = opposite of praise = scold

   After **chastising** Rex for the poorly written story, Gina felt so bad that she spent the next hour praising his writing skills.

   d. **Compare** or **contrast:**

   > saccharine = sickeningly sweet

   The sauce contained honey, but it was not at all **saccharine** like sugar-fortified syrup that Hal had poured on cake.

   e. Use the **situation:**

   Paula took a shot at the basket, but the ball missed badly, clanked off the rim, and **caromed** back to Paula.

   > **carom** = rebound

3. **Replace:** After you have settled on a guess, replace the unfamiliar word with your guess.

   > **Guess:**
   > **opulent** = luxurious

   The room was filled with **opulent luxurious** furnishings that were beautiful and clearly expensive.

4. If your guess makes sense within the context, your answer is likely to be correct.

3.4

Problem 2:

Which of the following is a synonym for the underlined word in this sentence?

The six-time Grammy winner started walking down the sidewalk and was soon <u>beset</u> by a mass of fans shouting her name.

A) helped   B) resisted   C) surrounded   D) lifted

STRATEGY

Refer to "situation" strategy in which you can use your real-world knowledge to make an intelligent guess.

THINK

- A famous person is walking down the street.

- The fans are shouting her name. They are unlikely to be helping her (A). They are coming toward her rather than resisting her, so (B) is incorrect. It makes no sense for the fans to be lifting the celebrity, so (D) is also wrong.

- This leaves (C) as the correct answer. The celebrity is being surrounded by her fans.

3.5 **COMMON ERRORS: *WHO* AND *WHOM, LAY* AND *LIE***

1. **Who** and **whom:** This is perhaps the toughest of all common usage errors. Don't be ashamed if you find *who* and *whom* difficult.

   a. *Who* is subjective—it takes the place of the subject of a sentence or clause, such as *he, she,* or *they.*

   b. *Whom* is objective—it takes the place of an object in a sentence, such as *him, her,* or *them.*

   c. So the best way to see which word should be used is to find the subject of the sentence or clause where it appears.

Subject: ***who***   Object (not the subject): ***whom***

Who is going to the store? (Subject: ***who***)

Whom do you trust? (Subject: *You,* so ***Whom*** is the object.)

Andrea, who is six, has two kittens. (Subject of clause: ***who***)

Mike, for whom I have great respect, made a big mistake. (Subject of the clause: *I,* so ***whom*** is the object)

   d. Prepositions always have objects, so they always take *whom.*

Dwight is the baker <u>for</u> whom the bakery was named.

2. **Lay** and **Lie**

   a. *Lay* is a verb that means to put down. It has nothing to do with reclining.

   b. *Lie* is a verb that means to recline as in something you would do on a bed.

Present	lay	I lay the pencil on the table today.
Past	laid	Yesterday I laid the pencil on the table.
Participle	laid	In the past, I have laid many pencils on this table.
Present	lie	Today I lie on the bed.
Past	lay	Yesterday I lay on the bed.
Participle	lain	In the past I have lain many times on this bed.

3. Note that the present tense of *lay* and the past tense of *lie* are the same word, *lay.* This is a source of much confusion.

3.5

Problem 1:

Which sentence is correct?

A) I don't know whom was present at the meeting.

B) I don't know who was present at the meeting.

C) Whom was present at the meeting?

D) I know who was present at the meeting.

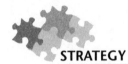

STRATEGY

Refer to the rules for each pair.

THINK

- In (B) and (D), the subject of the sentence was *I,* and *who* is the object of *know.* As the object, *whom* should be used rather than *who,* so both of these choices are wrong.

- In (C), the word *Whom* is the subject of the sentence, so *Who* should be used.

- These leaves (A) as the correct response. The subject of the sentence is *I.* The object of *know* is *whom,* so although it sounds awkward, (A) is correct.

- **Test tips:** When in doubt about *who* and *whom,* try to recast the sentence to avoid ambiguity.

3.5

Problem 2:

Which sentence is correct?

A) After being up for hours, the patient finally lay down and is now asleep.

B) After being up for hours, the patient finally laid down and is now asleep

C) After being up for hours, the patient finally lied down and is now asleep

D) After being up for hours, the patient finally has laid down and is now asleep

STRATEGY

Refer to the rules for each pair.

THINK

- The sentence is about being asleep, so it uses the verb *lie.*

- (B) and (D) both use *laid,* a form of the verb *lay,* so neither can be correct. (C) uses a verb form that fits neither *lay* or *lie,* so it is wrong.

- In (A), *lay* is being used in the past tense, so it is correct for this context.

Math

4.1 WHOLE NUMBERS AND NUMBER FACTS

A. Addition and Subtraction

1. All math begins with the four basic **operations**: addition, subtraction, multiplication, and division. Basic number facts are critical to these operations and for almost all mathematical operations.

2. If you do not have the basic number facts fully memorized and "automatic," take some time to learn them. An excellent learning method for number facts is to create individual flash cards and to drill yourself with them for a few minutes each day.

FLASH CARDS

8 + 3	11	13 − 6	7
front side	back side	front side	back side

3. Below are the basic **number facts**. To use the table, find the intersection of a row and column. For example, 6 + 7 = 13 is shown below.

Addition/Subtraction								
	1	**2**	**3**	**4**	**5**	**6**	**7**	**8**	**9**
1	2	3	4	5	6	7	8	9	10
2	3	4	5	6	7	8	9	10	11
3	4	5	6	7	8	9	10	11	12
4	5	6	7	8	9	10	11	12	13

	1	2	3	4	5	6	7	8	9
5	6	7	8	9	10	**11**	12	13	14
6	7	8	9	10	11	**12**	13	14	15
7	8	9	10	11	12	**13**	14	15	16
8	9	10	11	12	13	14	15	16	17
9	10	11	12	13	14	15	16	17	18

B. The Backward Relationship

1. Note that knowing an addition fact means that you also know the corresponding subtraction fact "backward." For example, if you know 3 + 6 = 9:

   $3 + 6 = 9 \rightarrow 9 - 6 = 3 \rightarrow 9 - 3 = 6$

2. Similarly, because 7 + 4 = 11:

   $7 + 4 = 11 \rightarrow 11 - 7 = 4 \rightarrow 11 - 4 = 7$

3. The basic "backward" facts work as a check on any **sum** or difference that you have calculated. For example:

   Does 90 − 34 = 56?

Check:

   34 + 56 = 90

4. Because the sum of 34 and 56 *is* 90, your answer checks.

C. Multiplication and Division

1. The basic multiplication and division facts are just as essential as the addition and subtraction facts.

2. Take some time to make some flash cards if you don't know these facts.

FLASH CARDS

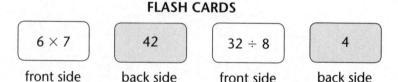

6 × 7	42	32 ÷ 8	4
front side	back side	front side	back side

Addition/Subtraction								
	1	**2**	**3**	**4**	**5**	**6**	**7**	**8**	**9**
1	1	2	3	4	5	6	7	8	9
2	2	4	6	8	10	12	14	16	18
3	3	6	9	12	15	18	21	24	27
4	4	8	12	16	20	24	28	32	36
5	5	10	15	20	25	30	35	40	45
6	6	12	18	24	30	36	42	48	54
7	7	14	21	28	35	42	49	56	63
8	8	16	24	32	40	48	56	64	72
9	9	18	27	36	45	54	63	72	81

3. The backward relationship works for multiplication and division as well as addition and subtraction. For example, if you know $8 \times 7 = 56$:

$$8 \times 7 = 56 \;\rightarrow\; 56 \div 7 = 8 \;\rightarrow\; 56 \div 8 = 7$$

As with addition and subtraction, multiplication works as a check on division, and division works as a check for multiplication. For example:

Does $426 \div 6 = 71$?

Check backward:

$71 \times 6 = 426$

Because the **product** of 71 and 6 *is* 426, your answer checks.

4.2 BASIC OPERATIONS

A. Addition

4.2

Problem 1:

Mountain climbers ascended 4738 m from their base camp at an elevation of 817 m. How high did the climbers climb in all?

A) 4555 m   B) 5545 m   C) 4545 m   D) 5555 m

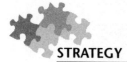

STRATEGY

The problem is asking for a total "in all" (see Solving Math Word Problems, Chapter 1.1). That means addition. For addition, line up the digits and add digit by digit.

THINK

- **Ones column:** 8 + 7 equals 15. Write the 5 below; then "carry" the 10 as a "1" above.

	¹4	7	¹3	8
+		8	1	7
	5	5	5	5

- **Tens column:** 3 + 1 carried is 4. Add 4 and 1 to get 5. Write the 5 below.

- **Hundreds column:** 7 + 8 is 15. Write the 5 below; carry the 1 above.

- **Thousands column:** 4 + 1 carried is 5. Write the 5.

- The sum of 4738 + 817 is 5555 (answer choice D). The climbers reached a height of 5555 m in all.

- **Check:** Subtract 817 from 5555 to check: 5555 − 817 = 4738

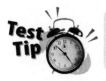

TEAS tests typically do NOT require "messy" calculations like this one. For most problems, simple calculations, mental math, estimation, and mastery of basic addition facts are sufficient for obtaining the correct answer.

B. Subtraction

4.2

Problem 2:

Elmville Memorial Hospital has 2002 beds. Hawthorne Hospital has 907 beds. How many fewer beds does Hawthorne Hospital have?

A) 2095　　　B) 2909　　　C) 1095　　　D) 995

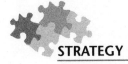

STRATEGY

The problem is asking for "how many fewer," so it uses subtraction (see Solving Math Word Problems, Chapter 1.1). Line up the digits and subtract 907 from 2002.

THINK

- **Ones column:** 2 − 7 can't be done, so a 10 must be borrowed.

- **Tens column:** The 10 can't be borrowed from the tens column, so move to the hundreds column.

	1̶	9̶	9̶	1̶
	2̶	0̶	0̶	2
−		9	0	7
	1	0	9	5

- **Hundreds column:** 100 can't be borrowed from the hundreds column, so move to the thousands column.

- **Thousands column:** Borrow 1000. Cross out the 2 and write 1 for the thousands column. Distribute that thousand over the hundreds, tens, and ones columns as 9 hundreds, 9 tens, and 10 ones.

- **Hundreds, tens column:** Cross out the zeroes in the hundreds and tens columns and write 9s.

- **Ones column:** Write the borrowed 10 into the ones column to make 10 + 2 = 12. Subtract 12 − 7 = 5. Write the 5.

- **Continue to subtract normally:** 2002 − 907 = 1095. Hawthorne Hospital has 1095 fewer beds. The correct response is (C).

- **Check:** Add 1095 and 907 to check: 1095 + 907 = 2002.

C. Multiplication

Problem 3:

Albuquerque averages 346 days of sunshine a year. How many total days of sunshine would Albuquerque have in 59 years?

A) 20,414   C) 18,554

B) 20,212   D) 24,140

STRATEGY

The problem is asking for a total that is a multiple of a single figure, so it involves multiplication (see Solving Math Word Problems, Chapter 1.1). Multiply 346 by 59 in two separate rows. Multiply the bottom row, 59, by the top row, 346.

THINK

- **Ones × Ones column:** Start at the right of the bottom number: $9 \times 6 = 54$. Write the 4 from 54 and carry the 5.

		²4̶	³5̶	
		3	4	6
		×	5	9
	3	1	1	4
1	7	3	0	
2	0	4	1	4

- **Ones × Tens column:** Continue with the 9 moving left: $9 \times 4 = 36 + 5 = 41$. Write the 1 from 41 and carry the 4.

- **Ones × Hundreds column:** Continue with the 9 moving left: $9 \times 3 = 27 + 4 = 31$. Write the 31.

- Cross out the "carries" and continue in the same pattern for the second line: 5×6, 5×4, and 5×3.

  $346 \times 59 = 20,414$.

- In 59 years, there would be 20,414 days of sunshine (answer choice A).

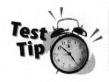

For any product, the digits in the ones column of the product must match the digits in the ones column of the factors. For this problem, the ones column digits of the factors, 6 and 9, have a product of 54, so the final product must end with the digit 4. That eliminates answer choices (B) and (D).

D. Division

4.2

Problem 4:

A stack of 37 books has a total of 15,503 pages. If all of the books have an equal number of pages, how many pages does each book have?

A) 409   B) 419   C) 4019   D) 4091

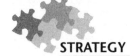

STRATEGY

The problem specifies items with an "equal number" of pages and asks for the size of "each" book. That identifies division as the operation being used (see Solving Math Word Problems, Chapter 1.1).

$$\begin{array}{r} 419 \\ 37\overline{)15503} \\ -148 \\ \hline 70 \\ -37 \\ \hline 333 \\ -333 \\ \hline 0 \end{array}$$

THINK

- Start at the first digit on the left. 1 divided by 37 can't be done, so move right. 15 divided by 37 can't be done, so move right. 155 divided by 37 is 4.

- Write the 4 in the **quotient**. Multiply 4 by 37 to get 148. Write 148 below and subtract.

- Continue the process until all digits are used.

- 15,503 ÷ 37 = 419. Each book has 419 pages (answer choice B).

- **Check:** Multiply 419 × 37 to check: 419 × 37 = 15,503.

4.3 ROUNDING AND PLACE VALUE

Rounding is a key method for estimation and mental math. If you need help in the decimal problems in this section, **see section 4.7,** Decimals.

4.3

Problem 1:

1. What is 2346 rounded to the nearest 100?

A) 2400   B) 2000   C) 3000   D) 2300

STRATEGY

Circle the **place value** you are rounding to; then look to the right.

THINK

- Because you are rounding to the hundreds place, circle the 3.

- Look to next place value on the right in the tens place. If the tens place digit is 5 or greater, round up. If it is less than 5, round down.

- The 4 in the tens place is less than 5, so round down.

thousands
hundreds
tens
ones

2 ③ 4 6
2 ③ 4 6
2 ③ 0 0

- Write zeroes in the places to the right of the number you are rounding.

- 2346 rounded to the nearest hundred is 2300. The correct response is (D).

4.3

Problem 2:

1. What is 19.796 rounded to the nearest hundredth?

A) 19.7   B) 19.80   C) 19.79   D) 19.8

STRATEGY

Circle the place value you are rounding to; then look to the right.

THINK

- Circle the place value you want to round to. Here, you are rounding to the hundredths.

- Look to next place value on the right.

- The 9 rounds up, so it turns to "10." Write a 0 and "carry" the 1 to the tenths place, turning the 7 into an 8.

tens ones tenths hundredths thousandths

1 9. 7 ⑨ 6

1 9. 7 ⑨ 6

1 9. 8 ⓪

- 19.796 rounded to the hundredths place is 19.80. The correct response is (B).

- **Key fact:** Always place a digit in the place value you're rounding to, even if it is a zero. The value 19.80 is different from 19.8 because it tells you that the number is accurate to the hundredths place, not the tenths place.

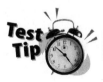

Test Tip

You can eliminate answer choices (A) and (D) because they are expressed to the nearest tenth, not the nearest hundredth.

4.3

Problem 3:

Which number is represented by DXCVI in Roman numerals?

A) 596   B) 546   C) 1096   D) 1546

STRATEGY

Identify the various Roman numerals. Work left to right.

THINK

- The D stands for 500.
- The X stands for 10. However, a C is placed to the immediate right of the X, so together XC makes 90.
- The V stands for 5. Adding an I (1) to the 5 makes 6.
- The sum of 500 + 90 + 6 is 596. The correct response is (A).

4.4 **ESTIMATING AND MENTAL MATH**

A. Using Estimation

4.4

Problem 1:

A rural bridge has a load limit of 6400 lb. A pick-up truck weighs 4324 lb empty. What would be the largest load that the truck could carry safely on the bridge?

A) 2100 lb   B) 2000 lb   C) 2050 lb   D) 2150 lb

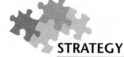

STRATEGY

You don't need an exact answer for this problem. You can use **estimation** to find a sum that is safely less than 6400 lb.

THINK

- 4324 lb is roughly 4300 lb. Adding 2000 to 4300 gives you 6300, well under the load limit, so you can eliminate 2000.

- Adding 2100 to 4324 puts you over 6400, so you know that both 2100 and 2150 are too high.

- That leaves 2050 as the answer (answer choice C).

B. Mental Computation

4.4

Problem 2:

The active ingredient in a dose of a drug has a weight of 7.6 mg. How many milligrams of active ingredient will 5 doses of the drug have?

A) 38.0 mg   B) 35.6 mg   C) 41 mg   D) 34.0 mg

STRATEGY

Use **mental math**. Multiply the whole number and the decimal separately.

THINK

- $7.6 = 7 + 0.6$, so:
$$5 \times 7.6 = (5 \times 7) + (5 \times 0.6)$$
$$= 35 + 3$$
$$= 38$$

- So 5×7.6 gives 38.0 mg (answer choice A).

4.4

Problem 3:

What is 300×16.3?

A) 480   C) 181

B) 489   D) 318

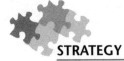

STRATEGY

Use mental math. Find the product of 1.63 and 100 mentally; then multiply the product by 3.

THINK

- $300 \times 1.73 = 3 \times (100 \times 1.63)$
  $= 3 \times 163$
  $= (3 \times 160) + (3 \times 3)$
  $= 480 + 9$
  $= 489$

> **Mental Math**
> $3 \times 16 \ = 48$
> $3 \times 160 = 480$

- So 300×1.63 equals 489. The correct response is (B).

☞ **Key fact: See section 4.7** on decimals for multiplying and dividing by powers of 10.

Test Tip *You know that 18.1×300 must be considerably greater than 300. This means you can eliminate answer choices (C) and (D) because they are far too small.*

4.5 INTEGERS AND NEGATIVE NUMBERS

A. Ranking

4.5

Problem 1:

Which of the following is the greatest number in this series:
−7, 0, −2.1, −0.8.

A) −7   B) −2.1   C) 0   D) −0.8

STRATEGY

When dealing with **integers** and **negative numbers**, think of a number line.

THINK

- Here are the four numbers from above on the **number line**. You can see that 0 is farthest to the right on the number line.

- So 0 has the greatest value. The correct response is (C).

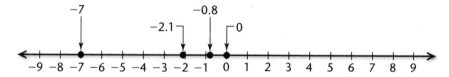

B. Adding and Subtracting Integers

4.5

Problem 2:

What is the solution to 5 − 8?

A) 3   B) −3   C) 13   D) −13

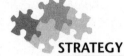

STRATEGY

Again, use a number line to visualize addition and subtraction on the number line.

THINK

- Move 5 spaces to the right to find 5.
- Move 8 spaces to the left to find −8.
- The sum is −3. The correct response is (B).

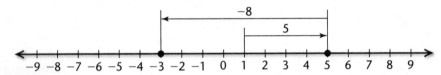

4.5

Problem 3:

What is the sum of −2 and −7?

A) −5   B) 9   C) −9   D) 5

STRATEGY

Use a number line.

THINK

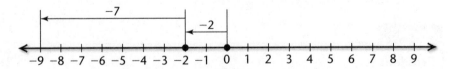

- Move 2 spaces to the left to find −2.
- Move 5 spaces to the left to find −7.

- The sum of −2 and −7 is −9. Answer choice (C) is correct.
- **Key fact:** You can use simple rules to add or subtract any two positive integers.

			Adding and Subtracting Integers		
Signs	**Order of Signs**	**What You Do**	**Final Sign**	**Examples**	
Same	++	Add	+	+3 + 5 = 8 +5 + 3 = 8	
Different	+−	Subtract	+ or −	+5 − 3 = 2 +3 − 5 = −2	
Different	−+	Subtract	− or +	−3 + 5 = 2 −5 + 3 = −2	
Same	−−	Add	−	−3 − 5 = −8 −5 − 3 = −8	

4.5

Problem 4:

What is the result of subtracting −6 from 4 as 4 − −6?

A) −2   B) 2   C) 10   D) −10

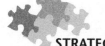

STRATEGY

In this case, you are subtracting a negative number.

THINK

- Write the problem: 4 − −6.
- Replace two **signs** with a single sign: 4 − −6 = 4 + 6 = 10.
- The sum is 10 (answer choice C).

C. Multiplying and Dividing Integers

4.5

Problem 5:

What is the product of −12 and 5?

A) 60   B) −17   C) −7   D) −60

STRATEGY

Multiply as you would normally. Use simple rules (below) to find the sign.

THINK

- Multiply the whole numbers: 12 × 5 = 60.

- Write the sign: −60. Answer choice (D) is correct.

Multiplying and Dividing Integers			
Sign	**Order**	**Final Sign**	**Example**
Same	+ +	+	+3 × +5 = 15
Different	+ −	−	+5 × −3 = −15
Different	− +	−	−5 × +3 = −15
Same	− −	+	−3 × −5 = 15

4.5

Problem 6:

What is the quotient of −84 ÷ −7?

A) 12   B) −12   C) −77   D) −588

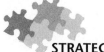

STRATEGY

Divide as you would normally. Use simple rules (above) to find the sign.

THINK

- Divide: $-84 \div -7 = 12$.

- Write the sign: 12. Answer choice (A) is correct.

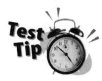

Just by looking at the signs, you know that the quotient must be positive. That rules out answer choices (B) and (C).

4.6 FRACTIONS AND MIXED NUMBERS

Fractions are a key to just about all types of math. Students who have trouble with other math topics, such as algebra or geometry, often can attribute a significant part of their difficulty to a failure to master fractions. So take some time to learn fractions (and mixed numbers). It'll pay off!

A. Ranking

4.6

Problem 1:

Rank these numbers in order from smallest to greatest: $\frac{1}{2}, \frac{5}{8}, \frac{5}{9}, \frac{2}{5}$.

A) $\frac{1}{2}, \frac{2}{5}, \frac{5}{9}, \frac{5}{8}$

C) $\frac{2}{5}, \frac{1}{2}, \frac{5}{9}, \frac{5}{8}$

B) $\frac{5}{9}, \frac{5}{8}, \frac{1}{2}, \frac{2}{5}$

D) $\frac{5}{8}, \frac{5}{9}, \frac{1}{2}, \frac{2}{5}$

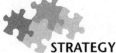

STRATEGY

Use models to visualize the fractions.

THINK

- Below are the fractions side by side.
- Draw a line to compare.
- So $\frac{5}{8}$ is greatest followed by $\frac{5}{9}$, $\frac{1}{2}$, and $\frac{2}{5}$, making answer choice (C) the correct response.

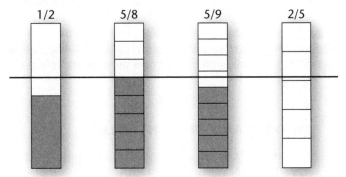

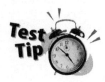

A good way to evaluate fractions is to compare them with $\frac{1}{2}$. In this problem, you can see that $\frac{2}{5}$ is smaller than $\frac{1}{2}$, and $\frac{5}{8}$ and $\frac{5}{9}$ are greater than $\frac{1}{2}$. That means you can eliminate choices B and D because they list $\frac{5}{8}$ and $\frac{5}{9}$ first in the sequence.

B. Greatest Common Factor, Lowest Common Multiple, and Simplifying

4.6

Problem 2:

Find the **greatest common factor (GCF)** for 18 and 24.

A) 4   B) 9   C) 12   D) 6

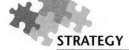

STRATEGY

Find the greatest number by which both 18 and 24 can be evenly divided.

THINK

- Find the factors of one of the numbers.
  24: (24 × 1), (12 × 2), (8 × 3), (6 × 4).

- List the factors in order: 24, 12, 8, 6, 4, 3, 2, 1.

- Find the greatest factor that divides evenly into the other number:
  - 24 is not a **factor** of 18.
  - 12 is not a factor of 18.
  - 8 is not a factor of 18.
  - 6 is a factor of 18.

- So 6 is the GCF (answer choice D).

4.6

Problem 3:

Which fraction is equivalent to $\frac{32}{48}$?

A) $\frac{5}{8}$ B) $\frac{3}{4}$ C) $\frac{1}{2}$ D) $\frac{2}{3}$

STRATEGY

Use the GCF to reduce the fraction to **simplest terms**.

THINK

- List the factors of 32 in order: 32, 16, 8, 4, 2, 1.

- Identify the greatest factor that divides evenly into 48: 16.

$$32 \div 16 = 2$$
$$48 \div 16 = 3$$

- The GCF is 16.

- Divide the **numerator** and **denominator** by the GCF as shown.

- $\frac{32}{48}$ in simplest form is $\frac{2}{3}$, making answer choice (D) the correct response.

4.6

Problem 4:

Find the **least common multiple (LCM)** for 8 and 6.

A) 16   B) 2   C) 24   D) 48

STRATEGY

Find the lowest number that can be divided evenly by both 8 and 6.

THINK

- List the multiples of each number. Find the lowest multiple that is common to both.

- 6, 12, 18, **24**, 30, 36, 42

- 8, 16, **24**, 32, 40, 48, 56

- 24 is the first multiple that is common to both lists, so 24 is the LCM, making answer choice (C) the correct response.

C. Mixed Numbers and Improper Fractions

4.6

Problem 5:

Express $\frac{15}{7}$ as a **mixed number**.

A) $2\frac{7}{15}$ B) $1\frac{2}{7}$ C) $2\frac{1}{7}$ D) $\frac{22}{7}$

STRATEGY

Divide the numerator by the denominator.

THINK

- $15 \div 7 = 2 \text{ R } 1$

- Express the remainder over the denominator.

- Answer choice (C) is correct.

$$\implies \frac{15}{7} = 15 \div 7 = 2 \text{ R } 1 = 2\frac{1}{7}$$

- **Key fact:** Any number expressed as a fraction can be simplified by dividing the numerator by the denominator. This method works for ordinary fractions, fractions that include decimals, and complex fractions that include fractions in their numerator or denominator.

- **Check:** Convert $2\frac{1}{7}$ back to an **improper fraction** (see below): $2\frac{1}{7} = \frac{15}{4}$.

4.6

Problem 6:

Express $3\frac{3}{4}$ as an improper fraction.

A) $\frac{15}{4}$ B) $\frac{33}{4}$ C) $3\frac{6}{8}$ D) $\frac{4}{15}$

STRATEGY

Work backward from a mixed number to an improper fraction.

THINK

- Express whole number 3 as fourths:

- $3 = 3 \times \frac{4}{4} = \frac{12}{4}$

- Add the 3: $\frac{12}{4} + \frac{3}{4} = \frac{15}{4}$, making (A) the correct response.

- **Check:** Convert $\frac{15}{4}$ to a mixed number.

$$3\frac{3}{4} = 3 + \frac{3}{4} = \frac{12}{4} + \frac{3}{4} = \frac{15}{4}$$

D. Adding and Subtracting

4.6

Problem 7:

Find the sum of $\frac{1}{6}$ and $\frac{7}{10}$.

A) $\frac{13}{15}$ B) $\frac{8}{16}$ C) $\frac{1}{2}$ D) $\frac{26}{30}$

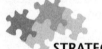

STRATEGY

Use the LCM to find the **lowest common denominator** for both fractions. Then add.

THINK

- Find the multiples:

- **6**: 6, 12, 18, 24, **30**, 36, 40

- **10**: 10, 20, **30**, 40, 50, 60, 70

- The LCD is 30.

- Multiply by a common factor to give each fraction the same LCD denominator of 30.

- Add the numerators to get a sum of $\frac{26}{30}$.

- Simplify $\frac{26}{30}$ to get a final sum of $\frac{13}{15}$, making answer choice (A) the correct response.

$$\begin{aligned} 1 \times 5 &= 5 \\ 6 \times 5 &= 30 \end{aligned}$$

$+$

$$\begin{aligned} 7 \times 3 &= 21 \\ 10 \times 3 &= 30 \end{aligned}$$

$$\frac{26 \div 2}{30 \div 2} = \frac{13}{15}$$

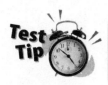

Test Tip

You know that $\frac{1}{2}$ (C) and $\frac{8}{16}$ (B) cannot be correct answers because $\frac{7}{10}$, one of the numbers you are adding, is greater than $\frac{1}{2}$ all by itself. That eliminates answer choices (B) and (C).

4.6

Problem 8:

Find the sum of $2\frac{3}{4} + 5\frac{5}{8}$.

A) $7\frac{3}{8}$ B) $8\frac{3}{8}$ C) $6\frac{1}{4}$ D) $7\frac{9}{8}$

STRATEGY

Add using the LCD; then simplify. Add whole numbers and fractions separately.

THINK

- The LCD is 8. (See above for LCD.)
- Express each fraction with the LCD.
- Change $\frac{11}{8}$ to $1\frac{3}{8}$ by dividing 11 by 8.
- Add $7 + 1\frac{5}{8}$ to get a final answer of $8\frac{5}{8}$, making (B) the correct response.

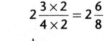

$$2\frac{3 \times 2}{4 \times 2} = 2\frac{6}{8}$$
$$+$$
$$5\frac{5 \times 1}{8 \times 1} = 5\frac{5}{8}$$
$$7\frac{11}{8} = 7 + 1\frac{3}{8} = 8\frac{3}{8}$$

4.6

Problem 9:

Rank the terms in order from greatest to least: $\frac{2}{3}, \frac{3}{5}, \frac{5}{6}, \frac{3}{10}$.

A) $\frac{5}{6}, \frac{2}{3}, \frac{3}{5}, \frac{3}{10}$

C) $\frac{3}{10}, \frac{5}{6}, \frac{3}{5}, \frac{2}{3}$

B) $\frac{2}{3}, \frac{5}{6}, \frac{3}{5}, \frac{3}{10}$

D) $\frac{5}{6}, \frac{3}{5}, \frac{3}{10}, \frac{2}{3}$

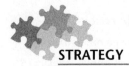

STRATEGY

Use an LCD to compare each term.

THINK

- List the multiples to obtain the LCM:
- **3:** 3, 6, 9, 12, 15, 18, 21, 24, 27, **30**, 33, 36

$$\frac{2 \times 10 = 20}{3 \times 10 = 30}$$

- **5:** 5, 10, 15, 20, 25, **30**, 35, 40
- **6:** 6, 12, 18, 24, **30**, 36, 42, 48

$$\frac{3 \times 6 = 18}{5 \times 6 = 30}$$

- **10:** 10, 20, **30**, 40, 50
- The LCM is 30, so use 30 as the LCD.

$$\frac{5 \times 5 = 25}{6 \times 5 = 30}$$

- Using the LCD, you can see that $\frac{5}{6}$ is the greatest fraction and $\frac{3}{10}$ is the smallest. This makes answer choice (A) the correct response.

$$\frac{3 \times 10 = 9}{10 \times 10 = 30}$$

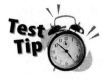

Test Tip

You can see that $\frac{3}{10}$ is the only term less than $\frac{1}{2}$, so the correct answer must feature $\frac{3}{10}$ as the smallest term. This eliminates answer choices (C) and (D) as correct choices.

E. Multiplying and Dividing

4.6

Problem 10:

Find $\frac{1}{6}$ of 72.

A) 16   B) $\frac{6}{72}$ C) 12   D) $6\frac{6}{12}$

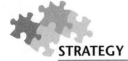

STRATEGY

Change both terms to fractions and multiply.

THINK

- **Key fact:** The key to multiplying or dividing fractions is to "cancel" by simplifying numerators and denominators as you proceed.

- Write each term as a fraction.
$$\frac{1}{6} \times \frac{72}{1} = \frac{12}{1}$$

- Use the GCF to simplify, much as you would when simplifying to lowest terms.

- Cross out terms that are simplified and replace them with the new values.
$$\frac{1}{\cancel{6}} \times \frac{\cancel{72}^{12}}{1} = \frac{12}{1}$$

- When fully simplified, multiply numerator by numerator and denominator by denominator:
$\frac{1}{6} \times \frac{72}{1} = \frac{1}{1} \times \frac{12}{1} = 12$. So (C) is correct.

- **Key fact:** When dealing with fractions and whole numbers in the same problem, it is best to convert all terms to fractions. Note that any whole number such as 72 or 117 can be expressed as a fraction by writing 1 as the denominator:

  - $72 = \frac{72}{1}$
  - $117 = \frac{117}{1}$

4.6

Problem 11:

Use mental math to find $\frac{5}{8}$ of 160.

A) 20   B) 100   C) 144   D) 96

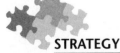

STRATEGY

Find $\frac{1}{8}$ of 160; then multiply that quantity by 5.

THINK

- **Key fact** To find a unit fraction of a quantity, such as $\frac{1}{3}$, $\frac{1}{4}$, $\frac{1}{5}$, or $\frac{1}{8}$, simply divide by the denominator. So $\frac{1}{8}$ of 160 is $160 \div 8 = 20$.

$$\Rightarrow 160 \div 8 = 20$$
$$20 \times 5 = 100$$

- Multiply 20 by 5 to obtain $\frac{5}{8}$ of 160, giving 100 for the answer. The correct response is (B).

Test Tip

You know that $\frac{5}{8}$ must be a little bit more than half of 160. That eliminates answer choices (A) and (C).

4.6

Problem 12:

Find the product: $\frac{8}{25} \times \frac{15}{16}$.

A) $4\frac{3}{5}$ B) $\frac{120}{400}$ C) $\frac{6}{20}$ D) $\frac{3}{10}$

STRATEGY

Use canceling to multiply.

THINK

- Use the GCF to simplify; then multiply.

- After multiplying, check your answer to make sure that it is in lowest terms.

$$\Rightarrow \frac{\overset{1}{\cancel{8}}}{\underset{5}{\cancel{25}}} \times \frac{\overset{3}{\cancel{15}}}{\underset{2}{\cancel{16}}} = \frac{3}{10}$$

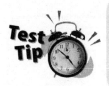

- *Answer choices (B) and (C) can be eliminated because they are not in lowest terms.*
- *Choice (A) can be eliminated because it is a mixed number—greater than 1. You should recognize that multiplying a fraction by a fraction will always result in a product that is less, not greater than 1.*

4.6

Problem 13:

Find the quotient: $\frac{7}{36} \div \frac{28}{45}$.

A) $\frac{3}{5}$ B) $\frac{120}{400}$ C) $\frac{6}{20}$ D) $\frac{3}{10}$

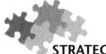

STRATEGY

To divide fractions, invert the **divisor** (the number you are dividing by) and multiply.

THINK

- Use the GCF to simplify; then multiply.

$$\frac{7}{36} \div \frac{28}{45} = \quad \text{divisor}$$

$$\downarrow \quad \downarrow$$

- After multiplying, check your answer to make sure that it is in lowest terms.

- $\frac{7}{36} \div \frac{28}{45} = \frac{3}{10}$

  The correct response is (D).

$$\text{invert}$$
$$\frac{{}^{1}7}{36_{5}} \times \frac{{}^{3}45}{28_{4}} = \frac{3}{10}$$

- **Key fact:** Dealing with fractions shows you that there is little difference between multiplication and division. Essentially, the two operations are identical except that in multiplication, you multiply by the fraction itself, but in division, you multiply by the inverse of the fraction.

4.6

Problem 14:

Find the product in simplest terms: $4\frac{3}{8} \times 1\frac{11}{21}$.

A) $6\frac{2}{3}$ B) $\frac{33}{168}$ C) $\frac{22}{3}$ D) $\frac{3}{20}$

STRATEGY

Change each mixed number to a fraction; then multiply.

THINK

- Use the GCF, if possible, to simplify.

- After multiplying, check your answer to make sure that it is in lowest terms.

$$4\frac{3}{8} = \frac{35}{8} \qquad 2\frac{11}{21} = \frac{32}{21}$$

- **Simplifying:** Note that 8 and 32 get cancelled and replaced by 1 and 4 because 8 divides evenly into 32 as 4.

$$\frac{\overset{5}{\cancel{35}}}{\underset{1}{\cancel{8}}} \times \frac{\overset{4}{\cancel{32}}}{\underset{3}{\cancel{21}}} = \frac{20}{3} = 6\frac{2}{3}$$

- **Simplifying:** Similarly, 35 and 21 get cancelled and replaced by 5 and 3 because 7 divides evenly into 35 and 21.

- The product of $4\frac{3}{8}$ and $2\frac{11}{21}$ is $6\frac{2}{3}$ (answer choice A).

4.6

Problem 15:

When you multiply 12 by a _____, the product is always _____ than 12.

A) whole number; smaller   C) fraction; smaller

B) fraction; greater   D) mixed number; smaller

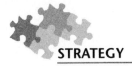

STRATEGY

Use a simple model to test your answer.

THINK

- Try multiplying 12 by a whole number. You get a product that is *greater* than 12.

$$12 \times 5 = 60$$ whole number: greater

$$12 \times 1\frac{1}{2} = 18$$ mixed number: greater

$$12 \times \frac{2}{3} = 8$$ fraction: smaller

- Try multiplying 12 by a mixed number. You get a product that is *greater* than 12.

- Try multiplying 12 by a fraction. You get a product that is *less* than 12.

- **Conclusion:** Multiplying by a fraction gives a product that is less than the number you are multiplying. Multiplying by a whole number or mixed number gives a product that is greater than the number you are multiplying. This makes answer choice (C) the correct response.

Quick Tips: Fractions

- Quick common denominator: Multiply the two denominators. What you get will be a common denominator but not the *lowest* common denominator (LCD). Example: For $\frac{3}{5} + \frac{5}{7}$: 5 x 7 = 35. Use 35 as a common denominator.

- Greater or smaller than $\frac{1}{2}$? Double the numerator. If the doubled total is greater than the denominator, the fraction is greater than $\frac{1}{2}$. If less, the fraction is less than $\frac{1}{2}$. Example: $\frac{5}{12}$: 5 x 2 = 10, which is less than 12, so $\frac{5}{12}$ is less than $\frac{1}{2}$. Example: $\frac{4}{7}$: 4 x 2 = 8, which is greater than 7, so $\frac{4}{7}$ is greater than $\frac{1}{2}$.

Divisibility Rules for Simplifying

- Divisible by 2: All even numbers

- Divisible by 3: Sum of the digits is divisible by 3.
  Example: 543: Sum of digits: $5 + 4 + 3 = 12$. 12 is divisible by 3, so 543 is divisible by 3.

- Divisible by 4: Sum of final 2 digits is divisible by 4.
  Example: 324: 24 is divisible by 4, so 324 is divisible by 4.

- Divisible by 5: The number ends with 5 or 0.

- Divisible by 6: Divisible by both 2 and 3 (see above)

- Divisible by 9: Sum of the digits is divisible by 9.
  Example: 495: Sum of digits: $4 + 9 + 5 = 18$. 18 is divisible by 9, so 495 is divisible by 9.

4.7 DECIMALS

A. Place Value

4.7

Problem 1:

Write the decimal number 0.016 as a fraction.

A) $\dfrac{16}{100}$ B) $\dfrac{1.6}{1000}$ C) $\dfrac{16}{1000}$ D) $\dfrac{3}{80}$

STRATEGY

Place value tells you how to write the fraction.

THINK

- The digit farthest to the right tells you the place value.

- The 6 is in the thousandths place. So the denominator of the fraction should be 1000.

- Write the numerator of 16 into the fraction giving you $\frac{16}{1000}$ (answer choice C).

hundreds	tens	ones		tenths	hundredths	thousandths	10 thousandths	100 thousandths	
0	0	.		0	1	6			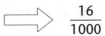 $\dfrac{16}{1000}$

4.7

Problem 2:

Write the fraction $40\frac{31}{10,000}$ as a decimal number.

A) 40.31   B) 40.031   C) 40.0031   D) 40.00031

STRATEGY

Use a place value frame.

THINK

- The denominator is 10,000, so write the 1 in the ten thousandths place.

hundreds	tens	ones		tenths	hundredths	thousandths	10 thousandths	100 thousandths
	4	0	.	0	0	3	1	

- Write a 3 to the left of the 1.

- Fill in the tens and ones places with 4 and 0, respectively.

- The tenths and hundredths have no digit, so fill them in with zeroes. So $40\frac{31}{10,000} = 40.0031$. The correct response is (C).

4.7

Problem 3:

Write the numbers in order from greatest to least: 0.2, 0.15, 0.34, 0.305.

A) 0.305, 0.34, 0.15, 0.2   C) 0.2, 0.15, 0.34, 0.305

B) 0.34, 0.305, 0.15, 0.2   D) 0.34, 0.305, 0.2, 0.15

STRATEGY

Compare digits in place value farthest to the left. Insert zeroes to compare numbers.

THINK

- The greatest place value here is tenths.

- The greatest digit in the tenths place is 3 in both 0.34 and 0.305.

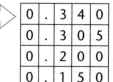

0	.	3	4	0
0	.	3	0	5
0	.	2	0	0
0	.	1	5	0

- Insert a zero at the right end of 0.34 to compare. You can see that 0.34 is greater.

- Insert zeroes to compare 0.2 to 0.15 and then 0.34 and 0.305. Again, you can see that 0.2 is greater. The correct response is (D).

B. Adding and Subtracting

4.7

Problem 4:

Find the sum of 165.093 + 6.8106 + 0.00057.

A) 228.9406   C) 171.90417

B) 185.90417   D) 0.17190417

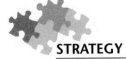

STRATEGY

Use a place value frame.

THINK

- Line up the decimal points. Write in digits as shown.

1	6	5	.	0	9	3		
		6	.	8	1	0	6	
		0	.	0	0	0	5	7
1	7	1	.	9	0	4	1	7

- Add as you would with whole numbers.

- Write the final sum 171.90417 (answer choice C).

- **Key fact:** Subtraction of decimal numbers is done in the same way: Line up the decimal points and subtract.

C. Multiplication and Division

4.7

Problem 5:

Find the product of 3.7 and 14.93.

A) 55,241   C) 55.241

B) 552.41   D) 55.421

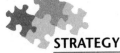

STRATEGY

Count the number of digits to the right of the decimal point. Multiply to obtain a whole number product; then count back to the left the same number decimal places.

THINK

- Count the number of digits to the RIGHT of the decimal point in both factors.

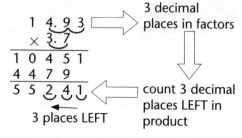

- Multiply as you would with whole numbers.

- Find the whole number product.

- Count the same number of places to the LEFT in your whole number product as you counted above.

- The product is 55.241. The correct response is (C).

4.7

Problem 6:

Find the product of 0.03 x 0.04 and compare it with the original factors.

A) The product, 0.012, is smaller than either 0.03 or 0.04.

B) The product, 0.0012, is smaller than either 0.03 or 0.04.

C) The product, 0.12, is greater than both 0.03 or 0.04.

D) The product, 0.12, is greater than 0.03 but less than 0.04

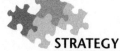

STRATEGY

Multiply as you did above. Compare the product with the factors that you multiplied.

THINK

- There are 4 places to the RIGHT of the decimal point.
- So move 4 places to the left to obtain a product 0.0012. Insert zeroes to hold places.
- Compare the product with 0.04 and 0.03.

$$\begin{array}{r} 0.0\ 3 \\ \times\ 0.0\ 4 \\ \hline 0.0\ 1\ 2 \end{array}$$

4 places RIGHT →

4 places LEFT ←

product	0	.	0	0	1	2
factor	0	.	0	3	0	0
factor	0	.	0	4	0	0

- You can see that the product is SMALLER than either factor (answer choice B).

4.7

Problem 7:

Moving the decimal point 2 places to the right in the number 6.2 is equivalent to which of the following?

A) Multiplying by 10   C) Multiplying by 100

B) Dividing by 100   D) Dividing by 10

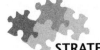

STRATEGY

Model using the number 6.2.

THINK

- Moving the decimal point 2 places to the right changes 6.2 to 620.

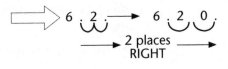

6.2 → 6.2 0

2 places RIGHT →

- As a check, try multiplying 6.2 by 10 and 100 and dividing 6.2 by 10 and 100.

$$6.2 \times 10 = 62$$
$$6.2 \times 100 = 620$$
$$6.2 \div 10 = 0.62$$
$$6.2 \div 100 = 0.062$$

- Clearly, moving the decimal point 2 places to the right is equivalent to multiplying by 100, making answer choice C the correct response.

- **Key fact:** Each decimal place that you move to RIGHT multiplies the quantity by 10. So moving 2 places right multiplies by 100, moving 3 places multiplies by 1000, and so on.

- **Key fact:** Each decimal place that you move to LEFT divides the quantity by 10. So moving 2 places left divides by 100, moving 3 places divides by 1000, and so on.

4.7

Problem 8:

Use mental math to divide 17.35 by 1000.

A) 0.1735   B) 0.01735   C) 0.001735   D) 1.735

STRATEGY

Dividing by powers of 10 can be done by moving the decimal point to the left.

THINK

- Each power of 10 moves the decimal point 1 place to the left.
- 1000 equals 3 powers of 10, or 10 x 10 x 10.
- So to divide by 1000, move the decimal point 3 places to the left.
- $17.35 \div 1000 = 0.01735$. The correct response is (B).

$$\implies 1\,7.35 \longrightarrow 0.0.1.7.35$$

$$\longleftarrow \text{3 places} \longrightarrow$$
$$\text{LEFT}$$

4.7

Problem 9:

Convert $\frac{5}{16}$ to a decimal number.

A) 0.3125   B) 0.516   C) 0.333   D) 0.165

STRATEGY

Divide the numerator by the denominator.

THINK

- Set up a division frame.
- Express 5 as a decimal—5.0. Write in zeroes to continue dividing.
- Keep dividing until the number divides evenly or you decide to round off.
- $\frac{5}{16}$ is equal to 0.3125. The correct response is (A).

```
        0.3125
16)5.0000
  -48
    20
   -16
    40
   -32
    80
   -80
     0
```

4.7

Problem 10:

Convert $\frac{25}{14}$ to a decimal number.

A) 1.667   B) 2.514   C) 1.786   D) 1.825

STRATEGY

Divide the numerator by the denominator as you did above. If the number does not divide evenly, round.

THINK

- Set up a division frame.
- Divide as above. Write in zeroes.

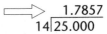
```
        1.7857
14)25.000
```

- Keep dividing. The numbers do not divide evenly, so round at the thousandths place.

- $\frac{25}{14}$ rounded to the thousandths place: $1.7857 = 1.786$ (answer choice C).

4.7

Problem 11:

Write the numbers in order from greatest to least: $0.7, \frac{2}{3}, \frac{7}{8},$ $0.801, \frac{5}{6}.$

A) $0.801, \frac{2}{3}, 0.7, \frac{7}{8}, \frac{5}{6}$　　　　C) $\frac{5}{6}, 0.801, \frac{2}{3}, 0.7, \frac{7}{8}$

B) $0.7, \frac{2}{3}, \frac{7}{8}, 0.801, \frac{5}{6}$　　　　D) $\frac{7}{8}, \frac{5}{6}, 0.801, 0.7, \frac{2}{3}$

STRATEGY

Convert all of the numbers to the same system, either decimal or fractions.

THINK

- Converting to decimal is usually easier than finding an LCD for all of the numbers.

- Change the fractions to decimal form as shown here. Round repeating decimals.

$$\begin{array}{r} 0.6666 \\ 3\overline{)2.0000} \end{array}$$

- Fill in zeroes to compare as shown below.

- 0.875 is the greatest value. 0.7 is the smallest.

$$\begin{array}{r} 0.875 \\ 8\overline{)7.0000} \end{array}$$

- Lining up the values shows that answer choice (D) is correct.

$$\begin{array}{r} 0.8333 \\ 6\overline{)5.0000} \end{array}$$

$$0.7000$$
$$0.6667$$
$$0.8750$$
$$0.8010$$
$$0.8333$$

4.7

Problem 12:

Find the quotient: 4.84 ÷ 0.08

A) 60.5   B) 6.05   C) 605   D) 0.605

STRATEGY

Move the decimal point to create a whole number divisor.

THINK

- Turn the divisor (0.08) into a whole number by moving the decimal point to the right 2 places.

- Move the dividend (4.84) to the right the same number of decimal places.

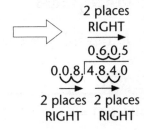

- Place the decimal point in the quotient (top) directly above the decimal point in the dividend.

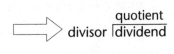

- Divide as you would with whole numbers. The decimal point will be correctly placed, giving a quotient of 60.5. The correct response is (A).

- **Key fact:** Use this frame to keep the names of terms *divisor, dividend,* and *quotient straight.*

4.7

Problem 13:

Simplify: $\frac{15}{0.6}$.

A) 9   B) 25   C) 90   D) 2.5

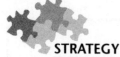

STRATEGY

Turn the fraction into a division problem.

THINK

- This fraction can be converted by dividing 15 by 0.6.
- Move the decimal point to the right 1 place to obtain a whole-number divisor.
- Move the quotient the same distance to the right. The quotient is 25 (answer choice B).

4.8 PERCENTAGES

A. Expressing Percent

4.8

Problem 1:

What is the decimal value of 3.5%?

A) 0.35   B) 3.5   C) 0.035   D) 0.0035

STRATEGY

Use the special "out of 100" ratio of percentages.

THINK

- **Key fact:** A percentage is a special ratio that compares a quantity to 100.
- **Examples:** 5% means "5 out of 100," 37% means "37 out of 100," and 62.5% means "62.5 out of 100."

- **Examples:** Percentages can also be expressed as fractions: 5% means "$\frac{5}{100}$," 37% means "$\frac{37}{100}$," and 62.5% means "$\frac{62.5}{100}$."

- **Examples:** Percentages can also be expressed as decimals: 5% means "0.05," 37% means "0.37," and 62.5% means "0.625."

- For this problem, you are going from 3.5% to decimal, so you divide by 100 to get 0.035 (answer choice C).

Ratio	Fraction	Decimal	Percent
1 out of 100	$\frac{1}{100}$	0.01	1%
5 out of 100	$\frac{1}{20}$	0.05	5%
10 out of 100	$\frac{1}{10}$	0.1	10%
20 out of 100	$\frac{1}{5}$	0.2	20%
33.3 out of 100	$\frac{1}{3}$	0.33	33.3%
25 out of 100	$\frac{1}{4}$	0.25	25%
50 out of 100	$\frac{1}{2}$	0.5	50%
66.7 out of 100	$\frac{2}{3}$	0.67	66.7%
75 out of 100	$\frac{3}{4}$	0.75	75%
90 out of 100	$\frac{9}{10}$	0.9	90%
100 out of 100	1	1.00	100%

Percent to decimal ⟶ ÷ 100

Decimal to percent ⟶ × 100

$3.5 \div 100 = 0.035$

4.8

Problem 2:

Express $\frac{5}{12}$ as a percent.

A) 51.2%   B) 5.12%   C) 41.7%   D) 62.5%

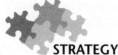

STRATEGY

Change the fraction to a decimal.

THINK

- Change the fraction $\frac{5}{12}$ to decimal form by dividing: $5 \div 12$.

$$\frac{5}{12} = 0.417$$
$$= 41.7\%$$

- To change a decimal to a percent, multiply by 100.

- $\frac{5}{12}$ is 41.7%. The correct response is (C).

4.8

Problem 3:

Express 65% as a fraction in lowest terms.

A) $\dfrac{4}{7a}$ B) $\dfrac{5}{8}$ C) $\dfrac{13}{20}$ D) $\dfrac{11}{20}$

STRATEGY

Change the percent to a decimal and then to a fraction.

THINK

- Change 65% to a decimal: 0.65.

$$65\% = 0.65$$

- Change 0.65 to a fraction: $\frac{65}{100}$.

$$0.65 = \frac{65}{100}$$

- Simplify $\frac{65}{100}$: $\frac{13}{20}$. The correct response is (C).

$$\frac{65}{100} = \frac{13}{20}$$

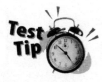

Test Tip

For this problem, all of the answer choices are "reasonable," so you should not make a guess based on estimation. Instead, this is one of the situations when you need to make a calculation. Note that the calculation itself is fairly simple and not "messy."

B. Three Types of Percent

Problem 4:

What is 45% of 120?

A) 45   B) 64   C) 54   D) 84

STRATEGY

Use one of the **three basic types of percent problems** as a model.

THINK

- **Key fact:** There are three basic types of percent problems that all fit the same basic framework.

- The framework has three variable parts: PERCENT, PART, and TOTAL.

- The PERCENT always has a percent sign, %.

- The PART precedes the word "is."

- The TOTAL follows the word "of."

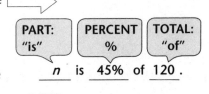

PART:	PERCENT	TOTAL:
"is"	%	"of"

$\underline{n}$ is $\underline{45\%}$ of $\underline{120}$.

$$\frac{PART}{TOTAL} = PERCENT$$

multiply both sides by 120

$$\frac{n}{120} = 0.45$$

$$\frac{\cancel{120}}{1}\frac{n}{\cancel{120}} = \frac{0.45}{1}\frac{120}{1}$$

$$n = 54$$

- The simple equation PART/TOTAL = PERCENT will solve any percent problem.

- For this problem, the TOTAL is unknown, so solve with: PART/n = PERCENT

- Multiply both sides of the equation by 120 to solve. This gives $n = 54$, making answer choice (C) correct. (Note: See section 5.2 for basic equation solving.)

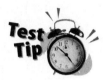

- *45% is slightly less than half, so your answer should be slightly less than half of 120. That rules out answer choices (B) and (D) because both are clearly greater than half of 120.*
- *For percent problems, you can use the equation method shown in this chapter or the proportion method in Chapter 5.*

4.8

Problem 5:

12.4 is 20% of _____.

A) 62   C) 2.48

B) 24.8   D) 124

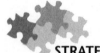

STRATEGY

Use the three basic types of percent framework.

THINK

- You don't know the "of" for this problem. So the TOTAL is the unknown.

- Place n in the denominator of the basic equation.

- Multiply both sides by $\frac{n}{1}$; then divide by 0.2 to isolate n.

- Solve: $n = 62$. The correct response is (A).

$$\underline{}\ 12.4\ \ \text{is}\ \ \underline{}\ 20\%\ \ \text{of}\ \ \underline{}\ n\ .$$

$$\frac{12.4}{n} = 0.2$$

$$\frac{n}{1}\frac{12.4}{n} = \frac{0.2}{1}\frac{n}{1}$$

$$\frac{12.4}{0.2} = \frac{0.2}{0.2}\frac{n}{1}$$

$$n = 62$$

4.8

Problem 6:

Last year, 128 babies were born on the fifth floor of the hospital. This year, 160 babies were born on the fifth floor. What was the percent increase in babies being born?

A) 20%   C) 25%

B) 28%   D) 16%

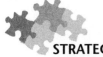

STRATEGY

Create a three basic types of percent framework comparing the increase with the original number.

THINK

- Find the increase:
  160 − 128 = 32.

  Increase = 160 − 128
  = 32 out of 128
  32 is *n*% of 128.

- Write a number sentence comparing the increase, 32, with the original amount.

  $$\frac{32}{128} = n$$

  n = 25%

- Write an equation.

- Solve for *n*: n = 25% (answer choice C).

- **Key fact:** Percent *increase* compares the difference with the original amount. Percent *decrease* compares the difference with the final amount. So to calculate the percent decrease here, you would compare 32 with 160, the final amount, rather than with 128.

Quick Tips: Percents

- Find 10% of a number: Move the decimal point 1 place to the left.

- Find 50% of a number: Divide in half.

- Find 1% of a number: Move the decimal point 2 places to the left.

- Find 25% of a number: Divide in half. Then divide in half again.

- Find 20% of a number: Move the decimal point 1 place to the left to find 10%. Then double that figure to make 20%.

- Find 5% of a number: Move the decimal point 1 place to the left to find 10%. Then find half of that figure to make 5%.

- 100% of any number is the number itself.

Algebra Topics

5.1 VARIABLES AND EXPRESSIONS

A. Simplifying Expressions

5.1

Problem 1:

Which expression is greater: $5 - (8)$ or $5(-8)$?

A) $5 - (8)$ is greater.   C) The expressions are equal in value.

B) $5(-8)$ is greater.   D) Both expressions equal -3.

STRATEGY

Remove parentheses; then simplify.

THINK

- Write the expression. Insert signs
  to give every term a sign.
- Resolve signs using simple
  rules (table below).

$$5 - (8) = +5 - (+8)$$
$$= 5 - 8$$
$$= -3$$

- Remove parentheses and simplify. -3 is greater than -40, so $5 - (8)$ is greater. The correct answer choice is (A).

$5(-8) = +5(-8)$
$= -40$

- **Key fact:** When there is no space between a number and a parentheses bracket, multiply. When a space exists, add or subtract.

Resolving Signs		
Sign	**Operation**	**Final Sign**
$++$	Add	$+$
$+-$	Subtract	$+$ or $-$
$-+$	Subtract	$-$ or $+$
$--$	Add	$-$

5.1

Problem 2:

Which of the following shows the distributive property?

A) $5 + 3 = 3 + 5$

C) $5 + (3 + 2) = (5 + 3) + 2$

B) $5(3 + 2) = 5(3) + 5(2)$

D) $5(3) = 3(5)$

STRATEGY

Identify the property where one term distributes over others by multiplying.

THINK

- Four different properties are shown in this problem.

$a + b = b + a$ (commutative addition)
$a(b + c) = ab + ac$ (distributive)
$a + (b + c) = (a + b) + c$ (associative addition)
$ab = ba$ (commutative multiplication)

- The **commutative** properties of addition and multiplication (answer choices A and D) show that a sum or product is the same backward or forward. For example, $6 + 4 = 4 + 6$.

- Answer choice (C) shows the associative property for addition, indicating that sums can be grouped in any order.

- Finally, (B) is the correct answer choice, showing that a term outside of parentheses distributes, or multiplies, over the terms inside of the parentheses.

- **Key facts:** One of the keys to algebra is the idea of the **variable**, a term that stands for a number or quantity, but has a value that can change. The letters a, b, and c above are variables. So are many of the x and y terms in the problems that follow in this chapter.

5.1

Problem 3:

Evaluate the expression $2x - 3y + 11$ if $x = 3$ and $y = -1$.

A) -16 B) 14 C) 20 D) -20

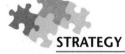

STRATEGY

Substitute value for each variable using parentheses.

THINK

- Write the expression.   ⟹ $2x - 3y + 11 =$

- Substitute the value for each variable using parentheses. $2(+3) - 3(-1) + 11 =$

- Simplify. The expression is equal to 20 (answer choice C). $6 + 3 + 11 = 20$

- **Key fact:** Make it a habit to use parentheses when substituting values for variables. Failing to use parentheses can result in confusion and mistakes.

- **Key fact: Order of operations** tells you the order in which to simplify a complex expression. The simplest way to remember order of operations is PEMDAS:

  P: Remove **p**arentheses

  E: Simplify **e**xponents

  MD: **M**ultiply and **d**ivide before you

  AS: **A**dd and **s**ubtract.

5.1

Problem 4:

Evaluate the expression $3 - 2(n^2 + 3) - 6n$ for $n=-5$.

  A) 13   B) –13   C) 3   D) –20

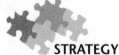

STRATEGY

Work left to right. Substitute values for all variables using parentheses. Then use PEMDAS.

THINK

- Write the expression.
- Substitute −5 for *n*.

$$3 - 2(n^2 + 3) - 6n =$$

$$3 - 2[(-5)^2 + 3] - 6(-5) =$$

- Remove inner parentheses first; then move to outer parentheses.

$$3 - 2[25 + 3] - 6(-5) =$$

- Take care of the powers: $(-5)^2 = 25$.

$$3 - 2[28] + 30 =$$

$$3 - 56 + 30 = -13$$

- Simplify until you are left with integers.

- The expression $3 - 2(n^2 + 3) - 6n = -13$ (answer choice B).

5.1

Problem 5:

Simplify the expression $3x + 2(x^2 - 5x) - (3x^2 + 4x)$

A) $11x - x^2$ B) $-x + 5x^2$ C) $4x^2$ D) $-11x - x^2$

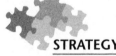

STRATEGY

Work left to right. Use order of operations and combine **like terms**.

THINK

- Write the expression.
- Remove the first parentheses by multiplying.

$$3x + 2(x^2 + 5x) - (3x^2 + 4x)$$

$$3x + 2x^2 - 10x - 3x^2 - 4x$$

- Remove the second parentheses by changing signs.

$$(3x - 10x - 4x) + (2x^2 - 3x^2)$$

$$-11x - x^2$$

- Regroup to simplify.

- Combine terms. The expression is equal to $-11x - x^2$, answer choice (D).

- **Key facts:** Terms can be combined (added or subtracted) only if they are **like terms**. Like terms have:

  o The same variable

  o The same power

In this problem $3x$, $-10x$, and $-4x$ were combined as like terms because they have the same variable (x) and the same power (first power). Similarly, $11x^2$, and $-x^2$ were combined as like terms because they both had the same variable (x) to the same power.

- **Key facts: Unike terms** can be combined only if they are multiplied or divided. Thus, in this problem, $2(-5x)$ gets multiplied to equal $-10x$.

B. Like Terms and Factoring

5.1

Problem 6:

The expression $5x - 10$ is equal to which of the following?

A) $-5x$ B) -5 C) $5(x - 2)$ D) $2(x - 5)$

STRATEGY

Combine like terms, if possible, or factor.

THINK

- Look to see if you can combine like terms. $5x$ and 10 are not like terms. They do not have the same variable and power, so they cannot be combined.

common factor = 5

$$5x - 10 = 5(x) - 5(2)$$
$$= 5(x - 2)$$

- Can $5x - 10$ be **factored**? It can if both terms can be expressed as products that have a common factor.

- Here we recognize that the common factor as 5: $5x = 5(x)$ and $10 = 5(2)$.

- We "factor out" the 5 from $5(x) - 5(2)$ using the distributive property in reverse.

- $5x - 10 = 5(x) - 5(2) = 5(x - 2)$, making (C) the correct answer choice.

- **Check:** $5(x - 2) = 5(x) + 5(-2) = 5x - 10$.

5.1

Problem 7:

Find the product: $(x - 5)(x - 4)$.

A) $x^2 - 9x + 20$ C) $x(x - 20)$

B) $x^2 - 1x + 20$ D) $2x^2 - 20x - 9$

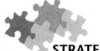

STRATEGY

Use the **FOIL** method to expand.

THINK

- The FOIL method stands for multiplying in this order: **f**irst, **o**uter, **i**nner, and **l**ast terms.

- The FOIL method is an extension of the distributive property in which you distribute by both terms, x and -5, in the first factor:

$$(x - 5)(x - 4) = x(x - 4) + -5(x - 4)$$

- The FOIL method is shown in the box below.

The FOIL Method

$(x - 5)(x - 4) = (x - 5)(x - 4)$ F *Multiply the first terms. Result:* x^2

$= (x - 5)(x - 4)$ O *Multiply the outer terms. Result:* $-4x$

$= (x - 5)(x - 4)$ I *Multiply the inner terms. Result:* $-5x$

$= (x - 5)(x - 4)$ L *Multiply the last terms. Result:* 20

$= x^2 - 4x - 5x + 20$

$= x^2 - 9x + 20$

- Note that you can use the FOIL method to expand any factors of the form $(a + b)(c + d)$.

5.1

Problem 8:

Factor the polynomial: $x^2 + 3x - 18$.

A) $x(x + 3 - 18)$ C) $(x - 3)(x - 6)$

B) $(x - 3)(x + 6)$ D) $(x - 3)(x - 6)$

STRATEGY

Set up a FOIL-type frame. Then find the factors.

THINK

- Look at the first term in each bracket first. You know that the first term in your polynomial is x^2, so it makes sense that x fits first in each bracket.

$x^2 + 3x - 18 = (? +/- \ ?)(? +/- \ ?)$

$= (x +/- \ ?)(x +/- \ ?)$

$= (x +/- \ 3)(x +/- \ 6)$

$= (x - 3)(x + 6)$

- Now look at second terms. The final term of the polynomial is -18, so you know the product of the terms is 18. The factors of 18 are 18, 9, 6, 3, 2, and 1.

- Ask yourself, "Which factors of -18 have a sum of $+3$ (to produce the $+3x$ middle term)?" You can see that 6 and 3 fit.

- Finally, the factors need to be different in sign in order to produce -18, and the 6 must be positive in order to produce a sum of $+3$. This means that (B) is the correct answer choice.

Check: $(x - 3)(x + 6) = x^2 - 3x + 9x - 18 = x^2 + 3x - 18.$

5.2 EQUATIONS

A. Basic Equation Solution Method

5.2

Problem 1:

Solve the equation $5x = 65$ for x.

A) 13   B) -13 C) $\dfrac{5}{65}$ D) $\dfrac{1}{13}$

STRATEGY

Apply operations to both sides of the equation to isolate the variable on one side of the equation.

THINK

- Write the equation.

  $5x = 65$

- Focus on isolating the variable. That means you want to remove 5, the coefficient of the variable.

  $\dfrac{5x}{1} = \dfrac{65}{1}$ multiply both sides by $\dfrac{1}{5}$

- To turn $5x$ into $1x$, multiply $5x$ by $\frac{1}{5}$, its **reciprocal**.

  $\dfrac{1}{\cancel{5}}\dfrac{\cancel{5}x}{1} = \dfrac{65}{1}\dfrac{1}{5}$

  $x = 13$

- If you multiply one side of the equation by a factor, you must multiply the other side by the *same* factor to keep things equal. So multiply the other side by $\frac{1}{5}$.

- Simplify $65 \div 5 = 13$, so $1x = 13$ (answer choice A).

- **Check:** $5(13) = 65$.

- **Key fact:** You can add, subtract, multiply, or divide an equation by any quantity—as long as you do the EXACT same thing to both sides of the equation.

- **Key fact:** The reciprocal of a number reverses the numerator and denominator. So for 8, the reciprocal of $\frac{8}{1}$ is $\frac{1}{8}$. The reciprocal of $\frac{5}{7}$ is $\frac{7}{5}$.

5.2

Problem 2:

Solve the equation $\frac{3}{4}n + 7 = 34$ for n.

A) $n = 28$ B) $n = \dfrac{1}{36}$ C) $n = 9$ D) $n = 36$

STRATEGY

Isolate the variable using both multiplication and addition.

THINK

- Write the equation.

- Working downward, subtract 7 from both sides of the equation to isolate the variable term.

- Express the result in fractional form.

- Multiply both sides by $\frac{4}{3}$, the reciprocal of $\frac{3}{4}$.

- Simplify $n = 36$ (answer choice D).

$$\frac{3}{4}n + 7 = 34$$

$$\underline{-7 = -7}$$

$$\frac{3n}{4} = 27$$

$$\frac{\cancel{4}}{\cancel{3}} \cdot \frac{\cancel{3}n}{\cancel{4}} = \frac{\overset{9}{\cancel{27}}}{1} \cdot \frac{4}{\cancel{3}}$$

$$n = 36$$

5.2

Problem 3:

A patient has been scheduled to receive 12 mg of morphine. The doctor has prescribed a maximum of 0.15 mg of morphine per kg of body weight for the patient. Is the 75-kg patient receiving too much medication?

A) No, the dose is just right.

B) Yes, the dose is 7.5 mg too high.

C) Yes, the dose is 0.75 mg too high.

D) Yes, the dose is 3.5 mg too low.

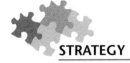

STRATEGY

Write equations to solve the problem.

THINK

- Label the maximum dose as m.

  Max dose $= m$

  $m = \text{wt} \times 0.15 \text{ mg}$

- Write an equation to find the maximum dose.

  $= 75 \text{ kg } (0.15)$
  $= 11.25 \text{ mg}$

- Compare the maximum dose with the dose that the patient is receiving.

  Overdose $=$ Actual dose $- m$

  $= 12 \text{ mg} - 11.25 \text{ mg}$
  $= 0.75 \text{ mg}$

- The dose of 12 mg is 0.75 mg more than what the patient is receiving (answer choice C).

B. Ratios and Proportions

5.2

Problem 4:

A nurse adds 4 g of salt to 20 ml of water to make a saline solution. How much salt should be added to 75 ml of water to make a solution of the same strength?

A) 0.25 g   B) 10 g   C) 15 g   D) 150 g

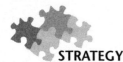

STRATEGY

Use a ratio and a proportion to solve the problem.

THINK

- **Key fact:** A **ratio** is a fractional relationship between two quantities.

- Here the ratio is 4 g salt: 20 ml water, or 1 to 5.

- **Key fact:** You can make a **proportion** by setting two ratios equal to one another.

- Here, we write *n* for the unknown quantity of salt.

  ratio $\quad 4:20 = 1:5 = \dfrac{1}{5}$

- An easy way to solve a proportion is by cross-multiplying as shown. You are left with a simple equation, $5n = 75$.

  proportion $\quad \dfrac{1\,\text{g salt}}{5\,\text{ml water}} = \dfrac{n\,\text{g salt}}{75\,\text{ml water}}$

  $$\dfrac{1}{5} \diagup\!\!\!\!\times \dfrac{n}{75}$$

  $$5n = 75$$

  $$n = 15$$

- Solve the equation in the normal way. The nurse would need 15 g of salt (answer choice C).

5.2

Problem 5:

Renay rode her bike 3.4 miles in 12 minutes. At this rate, how long will it take her to ride the entire 42-mile trip from her house to Santa Fe?

A) 157.5 min   C) 217 min

B) 1.57 hr   D) 2.57 hr

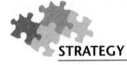

STRATEGY

Use a proportion to solve the problem.

THINK

- Renay's speed can be expressed as a ratio: 3.2 miles: 12 minutes. Express the ratio as a fraction.

- Set up a proportion using the ratio above and the 42-mile distance to Santa Fe.

$$\frac{3.4}{12} = \frac{3.2}{12}$$

$$\frac{3.2 \text{ miles}}{12 \text{ min}} = \frac{42 \text{ miles}}{n \text{ min}}$$

- Solve as you would normally. It would take 157.5 minutes to ride to Santa Fe, making answer choice (A) the correct response.

$$\frac{3.2}{12} \diagup\!\!\!\diagdown \frac{42}{n}$$

$$3.2n = (42)(12)$$

$$n = \frac{(42)(12)}{3.2}$$

- **Key fact:** In a proportion, make sure that units correspond. Here, for example, both numerators have miles, and both denominators have minutes.

$$n = 157.5 \text{ minutes}$$

5.3 MEASUREMENT

A. English (Standard) System

The system of measurement commonly used in the United States is the English system, which is summarized below.

Standard (English) Measurement		
Length	**Weight**	**Volume**
12 inches = 1 foot	16 ounces = 1 pound	1 cup = 8 fluid oz
3 ft = 1 yard	2000 lb = 1 ton	1 pint = 2 cups
5280 ft = 1 mile		1 quart = 2 pints
		1 gallon = 4 quarts

5.3

Problem 1:

How many feet are in 4.7 miles?

A) 24,000 ft   B) 2486 ft   C) 18,200 ft   D) 24,816 ft

STRATEGY

Use the conversion table above and a proportion to solve the problem.

THINK

- Set up the conversion using the number of feet as the unknown.

$$\frac{1 \text{ mile}}{5280 \text{ ft}}$$

- Solve.

$$\frac{1 \text{ mile}}{5280 \text{ ft}} = \frac{4.7 \text{ mile}}{n \text{ ft}}$$

- 4.7 miles is equal to 24,816 feet making answer choice (D) the correct response.

$$\frac{1}{5280} \times \frac{4.7}{n}$$

$$n = (4.7)(5280)$$

$$n = 24,816 \text{ ft}$$

5.3

Problem 2:

A nurse poured 3.2 quarts of liquid into a container. How many fluid ounces were in the container?

A) 96 fl oz   B) 44.4 fl oz   C) 102.4 fl oz   D) 202.6 fl oz

STRATEGY

Use a series of ratios to solve the problem. Cancel units.

THINK

- Write the quantity you want to convert as a fraction: $\frac{3.2\ qt}{1}$.

- Multiply your ratio by another identity ratio (from the table) that cancels with your units: $\frac{2\ pints}{1\ qt}$. Quarts cancel with quarts.

- Keep multiplying by different identity ratios until you reach the units you are looking for—in this case, fluid ounces.

- 3.2 quarts is equal to 102.4 fluid oz (answer choice C).

$$\frac{3.2\ qt}{1} = \frac{2\ pint}{1\ qt} \times \frac{2\ cup}{1\ pint} \times \frac{8\ fl\ oz}{1\ cup} = 102.4\ fl\ oz$$

- **Key facts:** Units are the key to conversion problems. Start with the units you have. Keep multiplying by identities to get to the units you want. Note: If the units of your answer are not correct, your answer cannot be correct.

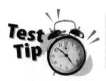

Test Tip

Use common sense and common knowledge to solve problems. For this problem, you may be aware that $\frac{1\ qt}{32\ fl\ oz}$. You can use this conversion identity directly to solve the problem rather than go through a series of conversions.

B. Metric System

The system of measurement commonly used in the United States is the English system, which is summarized below.

Metric Measurement		
Length	**Weight**	**Volume**
1000 millimeters = 1 m	1000 milligrams = 1 g	1000 milliliters = 1 ml
100 centimeters = 1 m	100 centigrams = 1 g	100 centiliters = 1 ml
10 decimeters = 1 m	10 decigrams = 1 g	10 deciliters = 1 ml
1 meter = 1 m	1 gram = 1 g	1 liter = 1 ml
1 dekameter = 10 m	1 dekagram = 10 g	1 dekaliter = 10 ml
1 hectometer = 100 m	1 hectogram = 100 g	1 hectoliter = 100 ml
1 kilometer = 1000 m	1 kilogram = 1000 g	1 kiloliter = 1000 ml

5.3

Problem 3:

45.6 cm equals how many hectometers?

A) 45,600 hm

B) 0.456 hm

C) 0.00456 hm

D) 4.56 hm

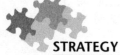

STRATEGY

Move the decimal point using powers of 10 to convert.

THINK

- Start with the units you want to convert: centimeters.

- Count the number of places you need to go to reach hectometers: 4 places.

- Move the decimal point 4 places LEFT to go from cm to dm.

  45.6 --> 4 places
  left = 0.00456

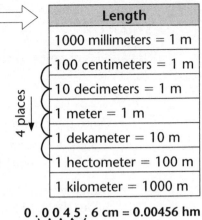

Length
1000 millimeters = 1 m
100 centimeters = 1 m
10 decimeters = 1 m
1 meter = 1 m
1 dekameter = 10 m
1 hectometer = 100 m
1 kilometer = 1000 m

4 places

0 . 0 0 4 5 , 6 cm = 0.00456 hm

- This means that answer choice (C) is correct.

- **Check:** A common-sense check for a conversion problem is of CRITICAL importance. 45.6 centimeters is about the size of your foot. So it must be a small fraction of a hectometer, which is 100 m in length.

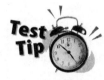

Test Tip

A centimeter, the size of your fingernail, is much smaller than a hectometer, which is longer than a football field. So you can definitely rule out answer choices A and D as far too large to be the correct answer.

Metric/Standard Conversion		
Length	**Weight**	**Volume**
1 km = 0.62 mile	28.35 g = 1 oz	1 liter = 33.81 fl oz
1 m = 39.37 in	1 kg = 2.205 lb	3.79 liters = 1 gallon

5.3

Problem 4:

Betsy has a 2.5-gallon jug of saline solution. How many ml does the jug contain?

A) 96 fl oz   B) 44.4 fl oz   C) 102.4 fl oz   D) 202.6 fl oz

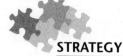

STRATEGY

Use a series of ratios to solve the problem. Cancel units.

THINK

- Write the quantity as a fraction: $\frac{2.5 \text{ gal}}{1}$.

$$\frac{2.5 \ \cancel{\text{gal}}}{1} = \frac{3.79 \ \cancel{l}}{1 \ \cancel{\text{gal}}} \times \frac{1000 \ \text{ml}}{1 \ \cancel{l}} = 9475 \ \text{ml}$$

- Multiply your ratio by another identity ratio (from the table) that cancels with your units. $\frac{3.78 \text{ liters}}{1 \text{ gal}}$.

- Multiply by other identity ratios until you obtain the units you are looking for—milliliters.

- 2.5 gallons of saline is equal to 9450 ml (answer choice C).

5.3

Problem 5:

Each day, a 125-lb patient is supposed to receive 0.8 mg of medication per kilogram of body weight. Which dosage should the patient receive?

A) 4.56 mg   C) 45.36 mg

B) 456.4 mg   D) 22.5 mg

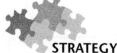

STRATEGY

Write equations to solve the problem.

THINK:

- Use a proportion to convert the patient's weight to kilograms.

$$\frac{125 \text{ lb}}{n \text{ kg}} = \frac{2.205 \text{ lb}}{1 \text{ kg}}$$

$$n = 56.7 \text{ kg}$$

- Write an equation to find the dose.

$$\text{Dose} = 0.8 \text{ mg} \times \text{wt}$$

- Calculate the dose.

$$= 0.8 \, (56.7)$$

$$= 45.4 \text{ mg}$$

- The patient should receive 45.4 mg of medication, answer choice (C).

5.4 DATA

A. Problems 1 to 3

The graph shows time allocation in hours for nurses on Floor 3 at the Sound Shore Hospital.

Sound Shore Hospital: Nurse Time Per Shift (hrs)

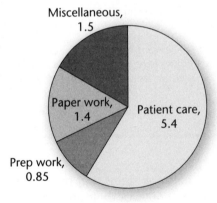

Miscellaneous, 1.5
Paper work, 1.4
Patient care, 5.4
Prep work, 0.85

5.4

Problem 1:

What percent of the time do nurses spend on prep work or paperwork?

A) 12% B) 38% C) 26% D) 58%

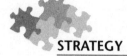

STRATEGY

Use the data in the graph and the proportion method of finding percents to solve the problem.

THINK

- Add to find the total number of hours in a shift: 8.65 hr.

  Total = 5.4 + 0.85 + 0.9 + 1.5
  = 8.65 hr

  Paperwork

- Find the total amount of time spent on paperwork and prep work: 2.25 hr.

  + prep = 1.4 + 0.85
  = 2.25 hr

  $$\frac{2.25 \text{ hr}}{8.65 \text{ hr}} = \frac{n}{100}$$

- Use a proportion to find the percentage of time spent doing prep work or paperwork: 2.25 out of 8.65 = 26% (answer choice C).

  $n=26\%$

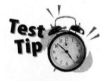

For percent problems, you can use the proportion method shown here or the equation method from Chapter 6, which is used in the next problem below.

5.4

Problem 2:

One nursing textbook states that nurses in a good-quality facility will spend at least 60% of their time in patient care, but in the best facilities, nurses devote over 70% of their time to patient care. What can you conclude about Sound Shore Hospital from the graph above?

A) The hospital rates as substandard.

B) The hospital is rated good but not the best.

C) Sound Shore rates among the best hospitals.

D) Sound Shore rates above even the best hospitals.

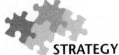

STRATEGY

Find the time in percentage devoted to patient care using the equation method of finding percents introduced in Chapter 6.

THINK

- Write out the equation as shown.

  5.4 is *n*% of 8.65.

- Find the percentage.

  $\dfrac{\text{PART}}{\text{TOTAL}} = \text{PERCENT}$

- Evaluate the percentage. Sound Shore qualifies as "good" because it is over 60% but not "best" because it is far less than 70%, making (B) the correct answer choice.

  $\dfrac{5.4}{8.65} = n$

  $n = 62.4\%$

The graph shows sanitation infraction records for Menlo Hospital over 3 months, showing incidents in which staff did not meet zero-tolerance sanitation standards for such things as hand washing, equipment use, protective clothing use, and so on. Use the graph for the following problems.

Menlo Hospital: Sanitation Infractions (per month)

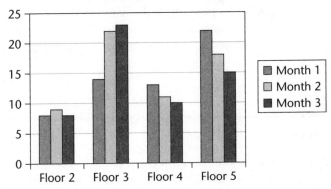

5.4

Problem 3:

Which floor showed the greatest improvement with regard to sanitation?

A) Floor 5   C) Floor 2

B) Floor 4   D) Floor 3

STRATEGY

Analyze the data in the graph and draw a conclusion.

THINK

- Note that the *fewest* number of infractions reflects the best safety record.

- Therefore, the floors that show a downward trend are improving.

- Both Floors 4 and 5 showed improvement. Floor 5 went from about 22 infractions to about 15, a greater decrease than Floor 4, so answer choice (A) is the correct response.

5.4

Problem 4:

Assuming sanitation and infection are related, on which floor would a patient have the smallest worry about contracting an infection in the hospital?

A) Floor 2   C) Floor 4

B) Floor 3   D) Floor 5

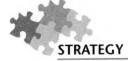

STRATEGY

Analyze the data in the graph above and draw a conclusion.

THINK

- Rather than looking at trends, look for the floor that had *fewest* absolute number of infractions overall.

- Floor 2, although not showing an improvement in its infraction record, nevertheless had the lowest number of infractions overall, so answer choice (A) is the correct response.

5.4

Problem 5:

Which floor showed the greatest percentage change with regard to infractions?

A) Floor 3 showed a 30% increase in infractions.

B) Floor 5 showed a 47% decrease in infractions.

C) Floor 5 showed a 32% increase in infractions.

D) Floor 3 showed a 64% increase in infractions.

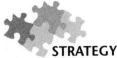

STRATEGY

Find the percentage change for the floor that had the greatest overall amount of change.

THINK

- From graph trends, it is clear that Floor 3 and 5 showed the most dramatic changes.

- Find the percentage change for each.

- Both floors had a large change of infractions, but Floor 3 had a change of 9 from its original 14, but Floor 5 went from 22 down to 15.

Floor 3 = 23 − 14
= 9 out of 14
$\frac{9}{14}$ = 64% increase

Floor 5 = 22 − 15
= 7 out of 22
$\frac{7}{22}$ = 32% decrease

- With a **64%** increase, floor 3 had the greatest percentage change, making choice answer (D) the correct response.

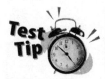

Test Tip

Keep in mind that percentage change always compares the change with the original number. Thus, in this problem, the change for Floor 3 was compared with Floor 3's smallest value, but the change for Floor 5 was compared with Floor 5's greatest value.

5.4

Problem 6:

The table shows scores in a gymnastics competition for Hector from six different judges. Which was greater, Hector's median score or mode score? By how much?

A) The mode was 0.15 greater than the median.

B) The mode and median were both the same, 8.6.

C) The mode was 0.15 less than the median.

D) The mode was 0.5 greater than the median.

Judge	1	2	3	4	5	6	7
Score	8.6	7.8	8.6	8.2	9.5	8.6	9.6

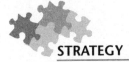

STRATEGY

Identify the mode and median in the data set. Then compare the two values.

THINK

- The **median** is the value that appears as the central value in the data set when it is arranged from least to greatest.

  Data set in order:

  7.8, 8.2, 8.6, 8.6, 8.6, 9.5, 9.6

  Median: central value

  Mode: most common value

- So 8.6 is the median.

- The **mode** is the value that appears most frequently in the data set.

- So 8.6 is the mode because it appears three times.

- The median and mode are the same for this data set, 8.6, meaning that answer choice (B) is the correct response.

5.4

Problem 7:

Which score change would push the mean value of the scores to 9.0 or above?

A) Judge 1 increasing her score to 9.5

B) Judge 2 increasing his score by 2.1

C) Judge 5 decreasing her score by 0.5 to 9.0

D) Judge 2 increasing his score to 9.5

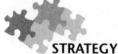

STRATEGY

The **mean** is the average score. Find the mean by adding to get the total of all scores and dividing by the number of scores. Find a score change that will result in a new mean of 9.0.

THINK

- Add to find the current total. Divide by 7 to get the mean: 8.7

  Mean: 8.6 + 7.8 + 8.6 + 8.2 + 9.5 + 8.6 + 9.6 = 60.9
  60.9 ÷ 7 = 8.7

- Now find the total that will yield a mean of 9.0

  Mean of 9.0: total ÷ 7 = 9.0
  $n \div 7 = 9.0 \longrightarrow n = 63$

- Finally, find the answer choice that gives a total of 63.0 or above. Answer choice (B) is the correct response. Increasing Judge 2's score by 2.1 gives a mean of 9.0.

  Judge 2: 7.8 + 2.1 = 9.9

  Mean: 8.6 + 9.9 + 8.6 + 8.2 + 9.5 + 8.6 + 9.6 = 63
  63 ÷ 7 = 9.0

5.5 ABSOLUTE VALUE, INEQUALITIES, RADICALS, AND AREA

5.5

Problem 1:

Solve: $|4x + 3| = 11$

A) $x = -2, x = 3.5$ C) $x = 2, x = -3.5$

B) $x = 2$ D) $x = -3.5$

STRATEGY

Set up two equations for the absolute value and solve each separately.

THINK

- The quantity inside of **absolute value** brackets is positive in all situations.

  $|4x + 3| = 11$

- Thus, for example, $|x| = 3$ has two solutions: x can equal 2 or –2 because $|2| = 2$ and $|-2| = 2$.

$$4x + 3 = 11 \qquad\qquad 4x + 3 = -11$$
$$\underline{-3 = -3} \qquad\qquad \underline{-3 = -3}$$
$$4x = 8 \qquad\qquad 4x = -14$$

- A more complicated equation works the same way: $|4x + 3| = 11$ is equivalent to $|4x + 3| = 11$ and $|4x + 3| = -11$.

$$\frac{\cancel{4}x}{\cancel{4}} = \frac{\cancel{8}^{\,2}}{\cancel{4}} \qquad\qquad \frac{\cancel{4}x}{\cancel{4}} = \frac{\cancel{-14}^{\,7}}{\cancel{4}_{2}}$$
$$x = 2 \qquad\qquad\qquad x = -3.5$$

- Solve each equation to find that $x = 2$ and –3.5, making answer choice (C) the correct response.

- **Key fact:** The absolute value brackets result in turning any quantity within the brackets to a positive quantity.

5.5

Problem 2:

Solve: $-5n < 15$

A) $n < -3$ B) $n > 3$ C) $n < -3$ D) $n > -3$

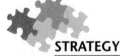

STRATEGY

Solve the inequality as you would solve an equation but flip the sign when multiplying or dividing by a negative.

THINK

- You can solve an inequality in the same way you would solve an equation except for one thing: multiplying or dividing by a negative will change the direction of the inequality.

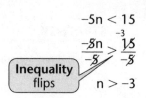

$$-5n < 15$$
$$\frac{-5n}{-5} > \frac{15}{-5}$$
Inequality flips
$$n > -3$$

- In this problem, you need to divide by −5. That flips the direction of the inequality from less than to greater than, making answer choice (D), $n > -3$, the correct response.

5.5

Problem 3:

What is the approximate value of $\sqrt{31} + \sqrt{20}$?

A) 51   B) 7   C) 10   D) 16

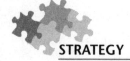

STRATEGY

Find the approximate value of each radical term and add them to find their sum.

THINK

- **Key fact:** The $\sqrt{\ }$ sign translates as "square root of" or "radical." For example, $\sqrt{16}$ means "the square root of 16" or 4 and −4. Similarly, $\sqrt{36} = 9, -9$.

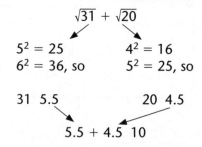

$$\sqrt{31} + \sqrt{20}$$
$5^2 = 25$ $4^2 = 16$
$6^2 = 36$, so $5^2 = 25$, so
31 5.5   20 4.5
5.5 + 4.5 10

- For $\sqrt{31}$, think of square numbers that are near 31.

- 5^2 is smaller than $\sqrt{31}$. 6^2 is smaller than $\sqrt{31}$. So $\sqrt{31}$ is between 5 and 6, about 5.5.

- Similarly, for $\sqrt{20}$, 4^2 is smaller than $\sqrt{20}$, and 5^2 is greater, so $\sqrt{20}$ is between 4 and 5, about 4.5.

- The sum of 5.5 and 4.5 is 10, making answer choice (C) the correct response.

5.5

Problem 4:

Find the area of the figure.

A) 526 cm²

B) 574 cm²

C) 696 cm²

D) 600 cm²

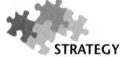

36 cm

12 cm

10 cm

16 cm

STRATEGY

Use the formulas for area of a rectangle and triangle to find the total area.

THINK

- First use the formula $A = l \times w$ to find the area of the rectangle: $A = 12 \times 36 = 432$ cm².

- Then use the triangle formula, $A = \frac{1}{2} h \times b$ to find the area of the triangle on the left. Use 12 cm as its height and 16 cm as its base: $A = \frac{1}{2}(12 \times 16) = 96$ cm².

- Use the triangle formula a second time to find the area of the triangle on the right. Use 10 cm as its height and 12 cm as its base: $A = \frac{1}{2}(10 \times 12) = 72$ cm².

- Add the three areas to get the total area: $A = 432 \text{ cm}^2 + 96 \text{ cm}^2 + 72 \text{ cm}^2 = 600 \text{ cm}^2$. This makes (D) the correct answer choice.

- **Key fact:** The height of a triangle is any length that extends from a corner to a side and forms a right angle. The base of a triangle is the side that the height intersects with a right angle.

Life Science

CELLS

A. Cell Types

1. All living things are composed of **cells**.

2. All cells come from preexisting cells.

3. All cells carry out the basic processes of life:

   a. Take in food and metabolize it for energy

   b. Respond to the environment

   c. Grow

   d. Reproduce

   e. Get rid of waste

4. All cells are one of three basic types that share a similar structure—prokaryotes, Archaea,[1] and eukaryotes.

Prokaryotes and Archaea	Eukaryotes
Single celled	Single-celled and multicelled
Bacteria, algae	Plants, animals, fungi, and protists
Extremely small cells	Large cells (10 times as large as prokaryotes)
No nucleus or organelles	Nucleus and organelles
Single circular chromosome	Multiple chromosomes
Reproduces by fission (budding)	Mitosis and meiosis (p. 184–188) for reproduction and growth

[1]Archaea are an obscure and recently discovered bacterial group that is different from the prokaryotes or "true" bacteria.

5. In addition to prokaryotes and eukaryotes, a fairly obscure third cell type is called Archeabacteria. All organisms belong to one of six **kingdoms**.

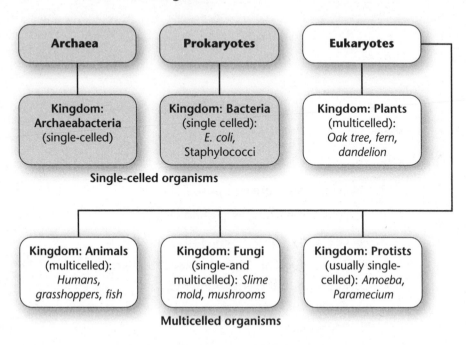

B. Cells in the Laboratory: Series Dilution of Bacteria

1. In series dilutions, a sample is repeatedly diluted. This series starts with bacteria of concentration c in the flask.

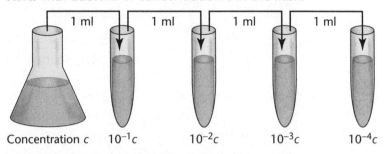

2. 1 ml is taken out of the flask and put into the first test tube with 9 ml of water, representing a 0.1 or 10^{-1} dilution.

3. The process is repeated three more times.

4. 1 ml is taken from the fourth test tube and found to have 40 bacteria.

6.1

Problem 1:

Which of the following is a characteristic of eukaryotic organisms only?

A) Forming tissues and organs   C) Cell division

B) Obtaining energy from food   D) Locomotion

STRATEGY

Refer to the characteristics of prokaryotes and eukaryotes.

THINK

- Both prokaryotes and eukaryotes carry out all of the basic life processes. So prokaryotes are capable of cell division (C), locomotion (D), and obtaining energy from food (B).

- Prokaryotes are not multicelled organisms, so they cannot form tissues or organs, making (A) the correct answer choice.

6.1

Problem 2:

Which life process is represented when you give off carbon dioxide when you are breathing?

A) Respond to the environment   C) Get rid of waste

B) Metabolize food   D) Reproduce

STRATEGY

Identify the basic life process that is carried out in exhaling carbon dioxide.

THINK

- Organisms take in oxygen and use it to "burn" food to obtain energy in metabolism. The waste product of metabolism is carbon dioxide. So when you exhale carbon dioxide, you are getting rid of a waste product. This makes (C) the correct response.

6.1

Problem 3:

A scientist views an organism in a high-powered microscope and sees that it has a cell wall and three separate chromosomes. What kind of organism is it likely to be?

A) Bacteria   C) Animals

B) Protists   D) Plants

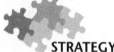

STRATEGY

Identify the characteristics of the kingdoms of life.

THINK

- The organism has a single cell, so plants (D) and animals (C) are ruled out. Bacteria (A) are single-celled organisms, but they have a single chromosome rather than multiple chromosomes. That leaves protists (B) as the correct response.

6.1

Problem 4:

How many bacteria transferred from the flask to the first test tube?

A) 4,000,000   C) 100,000

B) 400,000   D) 4×10^{-5}

STRATEGY

To solve the problem, work backward.

THINK

- Working right to left, each test tube has 10 times as many bacteria as the fourth test tube.
- Counting backward: $40 \times 10 \times 10 \times 10 \times 10 = 40 \times 10^4 = 400,000$.
- The original 1-ml sample transferred from the flask had 400,000 bacteria, making (B) the correct response.

6.2 CELL STRUCTURE

1. All cells have the same basic structure.

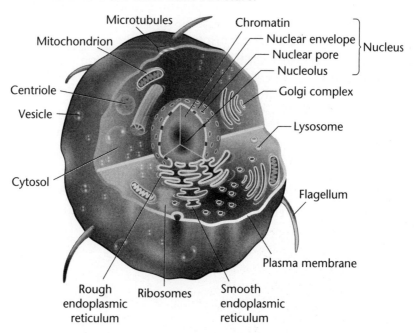

2. Eukaryotic cells have the **organelles**, or specialized membrane-bound structures. Note that prokaryotes don't have organelles.

Structure	What It Does	Who Has It
Nucleus	Regulates all cell activity; does this through DNA, which codes for protein enzymes that carry out all important cell "jobs"	All eukaryotes
Ribosomes	Use RNA to transcribe the original DNA code into proteins	All eukaryotes
Mitochondria	Cell powerhouses; use oxygen to burn glucose and produce ATP for cell's energy	All eukaryotes
Cytoplasm	Watery medium inside of cell	All eukaryotes and prokaryotes
Cytoskeleton	Provides structure for cell and allows for transport	All eukaryotes
Endoplasmic reticulum (ER)	Rough ER has ribosomes and produces proteins; smooth ER used in transport	All eukaryotes
Cell membrane	Barrier between inside and outside of cell; controls transport and water balance	All eukaryotes and prokaryotes
Cell wall	Stiff outer cell structure	Plants, fungi, and prokaryotes
Golgi bodies	Package proteins; secrete materials outside of cell	All eukaryotes
Vacuoles	Storage containers	All eukaryotes
Flagellum	Locomotion	Prokaryotes and some eukaryotes

6.2

Problem 1:

Which cell in your body would be likely to have a cell wall?

A) Skin cells   C) Bacterial cells in your gut

B) Liver cells   D) Neural cells in your brain

STRATEGY

Determine which kinds of cells have cell walls.

THINK

- Cell walls are present only in prokaryotes and among eukaryotes only on plants and fungi, not in animals. Therefore, human body cells such as liver cells (B), skin cells, (A), and brain cells (D) would not be expected to have cell walls.

- Prokaryotes do have cell walls, so bacteria, as prokaryotes, in the gut would have cell walls, making (C) the correct response.

6.2

Problem 2:

A patient has a cellular problem that involves protein synthesis. Which organelle would NOT be likely to be faulty?

A) Mitochondria   C) Ribosomes

B) Endoplasmic reticulum   D) Nucleus

STRATEGY

Refer to where proteins are made in the cell.

THINK

- Protein production is orchestrated in the nucleus (D) and carried out in the ribosomes (C), Golgi bodies, and endoplasmic reticulum (B), making all of these answer choices incorrect.

- The mitochondria are involved in metabolism, not protein synthesis, so (A) is the correct answer choice.

6.3 BIOLOGICAL MOLECULES

A. Key Molecules

1. All organisms have a number of key molecules that they use to carry out life processes. **Organic** molecules are those that include carbon.

Important Biological Molecules			
Molecule	**What It Does**	**Composed of**	**Examples**
Water	Life's "medium" Humans are about 70% water	Hydrogen and oxygen	Water
Carbohydrates	Energy source	Carbon, hydrogen, and oxygen	Sugars and starches
Proteins	As enzymes, proteins facilitate chemical reactions that are critical for life processes; structural proteins form muscles, connective tissue	Amino acid (see below) chains made of carbon, hydrogen, oxygen, and nitrogen	Pepsin (digestive enzyme), hemoglobin (red blood cells), and myosin (muscle cells)
Lipids	Fats; form cell membranes; used as an energy source	Carbon, hydrogen, and oxygen	Glycerol and triglycerides
Nucleic acids	DNA makes up chromosomes that code for all proteins	Carbon, hydrogen, oxygen, nitrogen, and phosphorus	DNA and RNA
Amino acids	Building blocks of proteins	Carbon, hydrogen, oxygen, and nitrogen	Lysine and glutamine

B. Nutrition

    1. The same molecules above are taken in as food and are keys to nutrition.

- Carbohydrates such as sugars and starches are broken down and "burned" for energy.

- Proteins in foods are broken down into amino acids and reformed into new proteins for muscle and other functions.

- Fats are burned for energy and used for building cell membranes.

    2. General diet advice includes:

- Maintain a diet of about 2000 calories. Growing, younger people may consume more. Older, less active people may consume less.

- Consume four or more cups of fruits and vegetables each day.

- Consume three servings of fiber-rich whole grains.

- Consume two servings of fish per week.

- Minimize intake of saturated fats and sodium.

- Consume four or more servings of nuts and seeds each week.

- Strictly minimize consumption of sugary foods, especially soft drinks.

    3. The diet goals above aim to support overall health goals that include:

- No smoking

- Healthy weight

- Regular exercise

- Manage blood pressure

- Control cholesterol

- Control blood sugar

    4. Vitamins are trace elements that are needed for good health. Note that taking vitamins in large doses can cause severe health problems.

Vitamin	Prevents	Food Sources
A	Night blindness	Yellow-orange vegetables, spinach
B$_1$: Thiamine	Beriberi	Pork, liver, eggs, potatoes
B$_2$: Riboflavin	Ariboflavinosis	Dairy, bananas, beans
B$_3$: Niacin	Pellagra	Meat, fish, eggs
B$_5$	Paresthesia	Meat, broccoli, avocados
B$_6$	Anemia	Meat, nuts, vegetables
B$_7$: Biotin	Dermatitis	Liver, egg yolk, peanuts
B$_9$: Folic acid	Birth defects	Leafy vegetables, liver
B$_{12}$	Anemia	Meat
C	Scurvy	Fruits, liver
D	Rickets	Fish, eggs, liver
K	Bleeding	Leafy vegetables

 6.4 **CELL STRUCTURE AND ACTIVITY**

A. Mitosis

1. Simple prokaryote cells (e.g., bacteria) have a single chromosome and reproduce by fission, which is similar to budding in plants.

2. Eukaryotes undergo **mitosis** for growth. The main purpose of mitosis is for the cell to accurately copy the DNA on its chromosomes and create new chromosomes for its "daughter" cells.

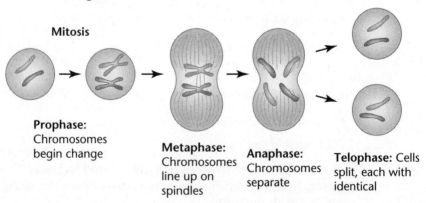

Mitosis

Prophase: Chromosomes begin change

Metaphase: Chromosomes line up on spindles

Anaphase: Chromosomes separate

Telophase: Cells split, each with identical

B. Sexual Reproduction and Development

1. In sexual reproduction, egg and sperm fuse to form a **zygote**, or fertilized egg.

2. Sperm are made in the testes, which are controlled by the hormone **testosterone**.

3. Eggs are produced in the **ovaries**.

   a. Each month, a single follicle matures and forms an egg or **ovum**, which is released from the ovary.

   b. The mature ovum enters the fallopian tube, where it may be fertilized by sperm to become a zygote.

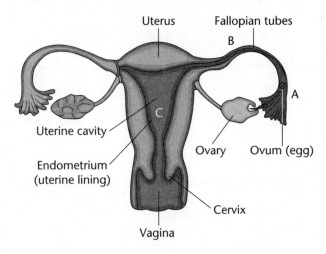

c. The zygote moves to the **uterus**, where it implants (in the endometrium) and begins to grow.

4. The growing cells undergo rapid mitosis and become an **embryo**.

5. If it fails to be fertilized, the egg will eventually dissolve within the fallopian tube. On the following month, a new egg will descend, and the process will begin again.

C. Meiosis

1. The goal of **meiosis** is to create special sex cells (gametes)—sperm and egg—for reproduction.

2. All ordinary nonsex "adult" cells MUST have two copies of every chromosome (2*n* or diploid).

3. If two "adult" (2*n*) cells with two copies of each chromosome were to fuse to form a zygote, the offspring would have four copies (4*n*) of every chromosome!

4. To avoid having too many chromosomes, organisms use **meiosis** to create special (1*n* or haploid) sex cells. Each sex cell gets only one copy of each chromosome (1*n*).

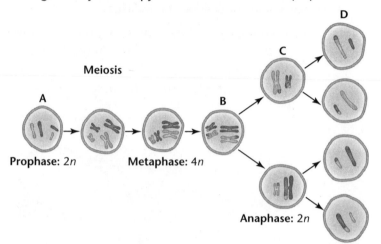

Meiosis

Prophase: 2*n*   Metaphase: 4*n*

Anaphase: 2*n*

Telophase: 1*n*

5. Now when two sex cells fuse, a 1*n* egg and 1*n* sperm form a new *2n* diploid individual. This individual has two copies of every chromosome.

D. Cell Transport

1. The environment of cells is dynamic. Small molecules are able to enter and leave a cell through its semipermeable membrane through the process of **diffusion**.

2. In diffusion, there is a net movement of materials from the place of higher concentration to the place of lower concentration.

3. When the cell is **hypertonic** to its environment, materials such as sugars, ions, and salts move out.

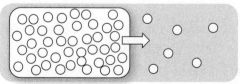

Hypertonic: Out

4. When the cell is **hypotonic** to its environment, materials such as sugars, ions, and salts move in.

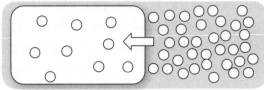

Hypotonic: In

E. Cells as Building Blocks

In multicellular organisms, cells are used as building blocks to form more complex body parts.

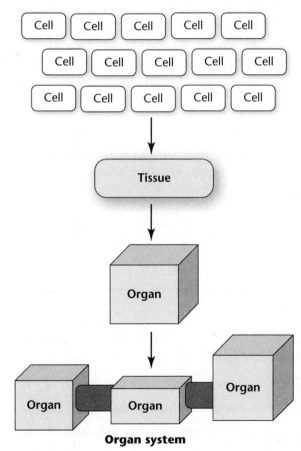

1. Cells joined together for a single function form **tissues**. There are four main types of tissue:

   a. Connective tissue (bone and cartilage)

   b. Muscle tissue (skeletal and cardiac muscles)

   c. Nervous tissue (brain cells, and spinal nerves)

   d. Epithelial tissue (organ surfaces, mouth lining, and skin)

2. Tissues join together to form **organs**. Examples of organs include the heart, brain, stomach, and kidneys.

3. Organs and tissues join together to form **organ systems**. There are seven major organ systems in the human body (**see section 6.5**).

   a. Circulatory system

   b. Digestive system

   c. Respiratory system

   d. Musculoskeletal system

   e. Nervous system

   f. Immune system

   g. Endocrine system

   In addition to these, other major organ systems include the urinary system, which controls excretion of cellular waste and maintains salt, water, and sugar balance within the body, and the reproductive system, which makes it possible for organisms to reproduce and have offspring.

6.4

Problem 1:

A gardener pours salt on a garden slug. What happens?

A) The slug expands in size.

B) The slug shrivels in size.

C) The slug doesn't change in size.

D) The slug's body shrivels while its head expands.

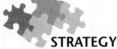

STRATEGY

Use the principles of diffusion.

THINK

- The slug has a proper water–salt balance for its environment to begin with. Pouring salt makes the slug hypotonic to its normal environment.

- To try to equilibrate, water rushes out of the slug. This causes the slug to shrivel, making (B) the correct response.

6.4

Problem 2:

An ovum stays in the fallopian tube for several days without moving. What can you assume?

A) The ovum is not mature.

B) The ovum has been fertilized

C) The ovum has not been fertilized.

D) The ovum may be twins.

STRATEGY

Refer to the steps involved in sexual reproduction.

THINK

- During the first stage of the cycle, the egg matures and moves to the fallopian tube. In the fallopian tube, the egg may or may not be fertilized.

- If it is fertilized, the egg will move on to the uterus. If it is not fertilized, it will stay in the fallopian tube and eventually disintegrate. This egg is not moving, so it must not have been fertilized, making (C) the correct response.

6.4

Problem 3:

As a normal human, Chuck has 46 chromosomes in his cells. How many chromosomes will Chuck's sperm cells have?

A) 46   B) 92   C) 184   D) 23

STRATEGY

Use the principles that underlie the ideas in meiosis.

THINK

- Sex cells fuse to form a zygote that has the normal number of chromosomes.

- If the zygote has the normal number of chromosomes, the sex cells must have half the normal number of chromosomes.

- This means that Chuck's sperm cells must have 23 chromosomes, half the normal number in his cells, making (D) the correct response.

6.5 BODY SYSTEMS

Body systems work together in a coordinated manner to maintain **homeostasis**, a stable environment inside of the human body.

A. The Circulatory System

1. The function of the **circulatory system** is to transport materials to and from the body's cells. Blood is the major carrier of these materials.

2. The materials that the circulatory system carries *to* the body cells include:

   a. Nutrients from the digestive system

   b. Oxygen from the respiratory system

   c. Hormones, such as insulin, that are secreted by glands and nerve cells

   d. Immune cells and products that fight infections

3. The materials that the circulatory system carries *away* from the body cells include:

   a. Waste products from cells that eventually get excreted as urine

   b. Carbon dioxide from cells that is eventually breathed out

   c. Excess salts and other materials that are often retained by the body

4. **Arteries** (red oxygenated blood) carry blood away from the heart. Arteries are thick and elastic.

5. **Veins** (blue deoxygenated blood) carry blood from body cells back to the heart.

6. The human heart has four chambers—**atria** on top and **ventricles** on the bottom. The left ventricle pushes oxygenated (red) blood through the aorta to the body.

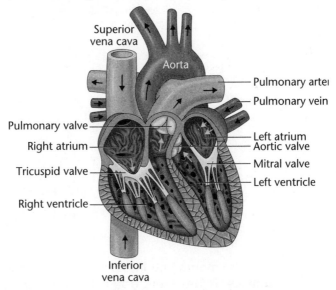

Superior vena cava
Aorta
Pulmonary arteı
Pulmonary vein
Pulmonary valve
Right atrium
Tricuspid valve
Right ventricle
Left atrium
Aortic valve
Mitral valve
Left ventricle
Inferior vena cava

7. Arteries branch into **capillaries**, where oxygen and nutrients get exchanged for carbon dioxide and wastes. Deoxygenated (blue, actually dark red) blood goes to the kidneys for cleaning and then back to the heart.

8. Blue filtered blood from the kidneys re-enters the right atrium and gets pumped from the right ventricle through the pulmonary artery to the lungs. (This is the only artery that carries blue blood.)

9. The blue blood exchanges carbon dioxide for oxygen in the lungs then re-enters the left atrium of the heart. From the left ventricle, this red blood is again pumped out to the body to begin the cycle again.

B. The Digestive System

1. The function of the **digestive system** is to break down food and deliver it to the circulatory system so it can be brought to body cells.

2. Digestion begins when mechanical chewing and enzymes begin to break down food in the mouth.

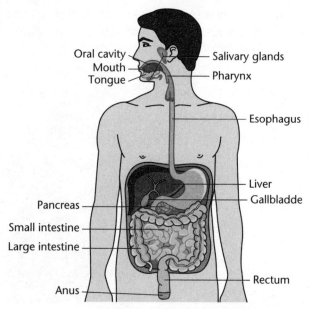

3. From the mouth, food goes through the esophagus to the stomach. Hydrochloric acid in the stomach of pH 1 to 2 (highly acidic) serves to kill bacteria rather than break down food. Mucus protects the stomach lining from this acid.

4. Food moves through the digestive system by the muscular squeezing action of **peristalsis**.

5. Enzymes work to break down food in the stomach. Then it is sent to the **small intestine** for further breakdown. Proteins are broken down into amino acids. Starches are broken down into simple sugars.

6. Fats are not soluble in water, so bile salts from the pancreas are secreted to emulsify them and break them down, much the way soap breaks down grease.

7. When broken down to the molecular level, food nutrients (sugars, amino acids, and small fats) get absorbed through the walls of the small intestine into the blood. The blood carries these nutrients to the body cells.

8. Indigestible food stays in the small intestine and gets passed on to the **large intestine**, where it is eliminated from the body.

C. The Respiratory System

1. The first function of **respiration** is to provide oxygen to the body cells for use in obtaining energy.

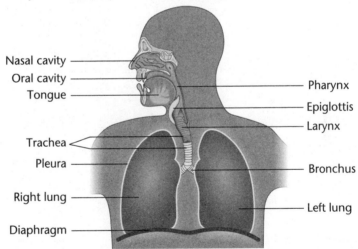

2. Oxygen and food in the body work in much the same way that gasoline and oxygen work in a car. A car needs air (oxygen) to burn gasoline to obtain energy. A body needs oxygen to burn food as fuel to obtain energy.

3. Nutrients and oxygen are delivered to the body cells through the circulatory system. The cells use the energy released from "burning" food to create the adenosine

triphosphate (ATP) that the body uses for energy (cellular respiration).

4. Heat is a byproduct of this combustion. Your body heat comes from the combustion of food.

5. As with a car or a fire, carbon dioxide is the waste product of combustion. Carbon dioxide is carried from the cells as "blue" blood and back to the heart.

6. Actual gas exchange takes place in the **lungs**. In tiny capillaries, oxygen is exchanged for carbon dioxide. Air and oxygen are breathed in. Carbon dioxide is breathed out.

D. The Musculoskeletal System

1. The **musculoskeletal system** includes the body's muscle system and its skeleton. The function of this system is to provide locomotion for an organism.

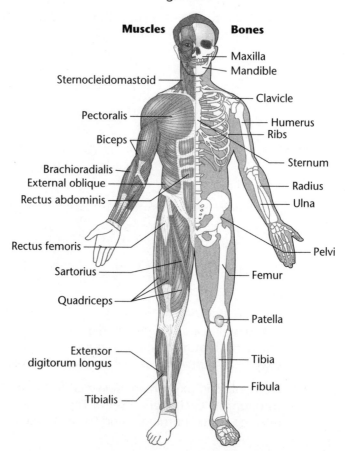

Muscles   **Bones**

Maxilla
Mandible
Sternocleidomastoid
Clavicle
Pectoralis
Humerus
Biceps
Ribs
Brachioradialis
Sternum
External oblique
Radius
Rectus abdominis
Ulna
Rectus femoris
Pelvi
Sartorius
Femur
Quadriceps
Patella
Extensor digitorum longus
Tibia
Fibula
Tibialis

2. There are three kinds of muscle tissue: skeletal muscle, cardiac muscle, and smooth muscle.

3. Skeletal muscles, which are attached to bones, are the only one of the three types that can be consciously controlled.

4. Smooth muscles move substances through organs. The digestive system has smooth muscles.

5. Muscles can only contract; they cannot extend.

6. Muscles are arranged in antagonistic pairs such as the biceps and triceps.

   • When the biceps contracts, the triceps relaxes and extends.

   • When the triceps contracts, the biceps relaxes and extends.

7. Bones are connected to other structures by tendons and ligaments. Whereas tendons connect bones to muscles, ligaments connect bones to other bones, usually at joints.

   Terms used in anatomy include:

   Superior: upper
   Inferior: lower
   Anterior: front
   Posterior: rear
   Medial: toward middle
   Lateral: toward outside

   Dorsal: back (as in a dog)
   Ventral: belly (as in a dog)
   Proximal: close, toward body trunk
   Distal: far, toward extremities
   Sagittal: lengthwise section
   Transverse: cross section

E. Nervous System

   1. The **central nervous system** (CNS) includes the brain and spinal cord and guides skeletal (voluntary) muscles.

   2. The brain and spinal cord control all thought and voluntary movement.

   3. **Neurons** (basic nerve cells) conduct information electrically along outgoing **axon** fibers and incoming **dendrites**.

   4. Communication between axon terminals and neurons is done chemically using **neurotransmitters** that are released into the synapse or junction between neurons.

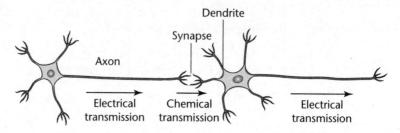

5. So information is conveyed both electrically and chemically. Axons and dendrites work like electrical wires. Synapses transmit information using chemicals (neurotransmitters).

6. In a voluntary movement:
   a. An electrical signal is sent from the brain to a motor neuron in the spinal cord.
   b. The motor neuron relays the signal to the muscle.
   c. At the muscle, the electrical signal gets transformed into release of chemical neurotransmitter, acetylcholine.
   d. Acetylcholine stimulates excitable muscle tissue to contract.

7. The peripheral nervous system, a network of sensory nerves that connect to the CNS, is divided into somatic (voluntary) and autonomic (involuntary) nerves.

8. Different regions of the brain are specialized for different functions.

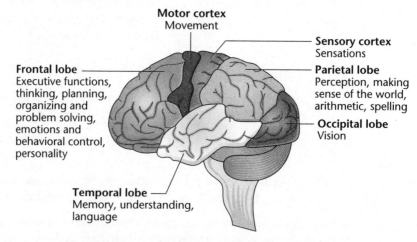

   a. The cortex, or outer "skin" of the brain, performs the most sophisticated functions.
   b. Visual information enters the back of the brain in the occipital lobe.

   c. Note that the sensory area is near the motor cortex for quick action.

   d. The "boss" of the brain is in the frontal lobe, where executive function and decision making largely occur.

F. Immune System

  1. The body has four lines of defense to protect against infections and **antigens** and pathogens (invaders).

  2. First, the skin and assorted body fluids (tears, mucus, saliva, waxes, and stomach acid) keep infections out and can expel them if they enter.

  3. Second, the swelling and redness of inflammation signal that the body has called in white blood cells and natural killer (NK) cells to consume bacteria.

  4. White blood cells (phagocytes) "swallow" bacteria (phagocytosis) that have been identified by helper T cells. Interferon is used to combat virus invaders.

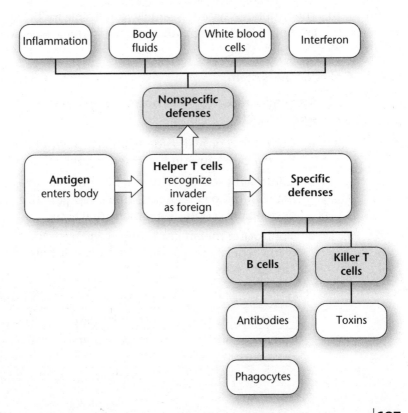

5. The body's third line of defense is specific—defenses are "custom made" to fight off specific infections. Antigens (foreign proteins) bind to **B cells**, which produce **antibodies** specific to that infection.

6. The immune system keeps a handful of antibodies around to "remember" a specific infection. If the infection shows up— even decades later—antibody production is quickly ramped up to fight off the invader.

7. With a **vaccine**, a weakened form of an antigen is introduced into the body to activate B cells to produce antibodies. If the nonweakened antigen then arrives, it is combated by the premade antibodies.

8. In the body's fourth line of defense, **killer T cells** rove the body seeking out "nonself" cells and mounting a campaign to kill them off.

9. Helper T cells help both B cells and killer T cells recognize invaders.

10. The lymphatic system is largely responsible for bringing antibodies and white blood cells to different parts of the body.

G. Endocrine System

1. The **endocrine** produces **hormones** or chemical messengers whose function includes:

   a. Controlling growth—for example, growth hormone from the hypothalamus in the anterior pituitary

   b. Controlling sexual development—for example, estrogen made in the ovaries helps female reproductive system develop and controls the menstrual cycle

   c. Controlling metabolism—thyroxine from the thyroid gland regulates basic metabolic rate, or how fast your "motor" runs

Hormone	Gland	Function
Growth hormone	Hypothalamus	Growth
Oxytocin and vasopressin	Hypothalamus	Uterine contractions

(continued)

(*continued*)

Hormone	Gland	Function
Thyroxin	Thyroid gland	Metabolism
Insulin and glucagon	Pancreas	Blood sugar
Cortisol	Adrenal cortex	Stress and metabolism
Estrogen and testosterone	Ovaries and testes	Sex

2. Hormones typically get secreted from a gland and travel through the bloodstream. When a hormone reaches its target, it changes activity, structure, or behavior.

3. Example: Insulin and diabetes

   a. When food is eaten and sugar (glucose) enters the blood, the pancreas releases **insulin** into the blood.

   b. Insulin allows cells to take in glucose. Without insulin, the body's cells cannot take in glucose.

   c. In normal people, blood sugar levels rise after eating and then drop as insulin is released and glucose is taken into cells and metabolized.

   d. A person with **diabetes** is unable to make insulin.

   e. Without insulin, the cells of a person with diabetes are "starved" for glucose. The person feels weak even though blood sugar levels remain high.

   f. People with diabetes must carefully control when and how much insulin to take so they can maintain healthy blood sugar levels.

H. Excretory System

   1. The key organs for the **excretory system** are the kidneys.

   2. Normal metabolism in cells produces waste products that enter the blue blood along with carbon dioxide.

   3. Before returning to the lungs for oxygen and the small intestine for food, this blood must be filtered and cleaned.

   4. Toxins are taken out of the blood in the liver.

   5. Filtering of waste occurs in the kidneys.

6. Kidney cells, or **nephrons**, feature a tiny **glomerulus** that acts like a filter.

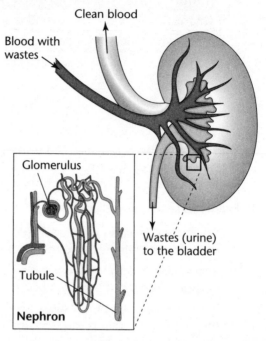

7. The glomerulus keeps proteins, key ions such as sodium and potassium, and other valuable substances in the body and allows waste and excess fluid to collect in a tubule.

8. This excess fluid and waste is ultimately excreted from the body as urine.

6.5

Problem 1:

Why is the pulmonary vein called a vein rather than an artery?

A) Because pulmonary vein carries blue blood

B) Because pulmonary carries red blood away from the heart

C) Because pulmonary carries blue blood to the heart

D) Because pulmonary carries blue blood away from the heart

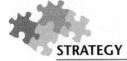

STRATEGY

Use the definition of arteries and veins.

THINK

- By definition, an artery carries blood away from the heart, and a vein carries blood to the heart.

- The pulmonary vein carries red blood that has just been oxygenated in the lungs. Because it carries blood *to* the heart, it is termed a vein rather than an artery.

- (A) is wrong because the type of blood that a vessel carries does not affect its name. (B) and (D) are incorrect because pulmonary vein does not carry blood away from the heart. (C) is the correct response.

6.5

Problem 2:

Where is food broken down in the digestive system so it can ultimately enter the bloodstream?

A) In the stomach

B) In the stomach, small intestine, and large intestine

C) In the mouth, stomach, and large intestine

D) In the mouth, stomach, and small intestine

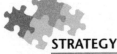

STRATEGY

Identify parts of the digestive system that break down food.

THINK

- Enzymes in the mouth begin the process of digestion. Digestion continues in the stomach, and food is broken down to its final molecular level in the small intestine. This means that (D) is the correct response.

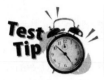

Test Tip

You should recognize right away that the food that enters the large intestine is not digestible and therefore is no longer broken down for absorption through the small intestine. This eliminates (B) and (C) as answer choices because both include the large intestine.

6.5

Problem 3:

What symptoms would you expect with a patient with low blood oxygen?

A) Joint pain

C) No symptoms

B) Weakness and low energy

D) Nausea

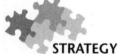

STRATEGY

Refer to the purpose of respiration to determine how low oxygen would affect a person.

THINK

- The goal of respiration is to supply oxygen to cells that is used to "burn" food and create energy in the form of ATP.

- Therefore, a person with low oxygen would be energy depleted and feel weak, making (B) the correct response.

6.5

Problem 4:

Which bone is proximal to the shoulder joint?

A) Radius   C) Ulna

B) Humerus   D) Femur

STRATEGY

Apply the definitions of *proximal* and *distal* to the bones shown in the figure on page 194.

THINK

- *Proximal* means close to the joint.
- The joint in question here is the shoulder joint. Both the radius (A) and ulna (C) are distal to the shoulder joint compared with the humerus. This makes (B) the correct response.

6.5

Problem 5:

A patient has been diagnosed with a chemical imbalance in his brain. Which part of his neurons is likely to be affected by this imbalance?

A) Dendrites   C) Synapses

B) Axons   D) Lateral

STRATEGY

Identify the part of the neuron that is most closely related to chemical transmission of information.

THINK

- In a neuron, the impulse travels electrically along the axon and dendrite, making (B) and (A) incorrect answer choices.

- When the electrical impulse reaches the synapse, it causes the release of chemical neurotransmitters that transmit the information to the next neuron in the sequence. This makes (C) the correct response.

6.6 BIOCHEMISTRY AND GENETICS

A. Photosynthesis and Cellular Respiration

1. **Photosynthesis** is the process by which almost all living things obtain energy.

2. In photosynthesis, plants use special pigments (chlorophyll) to convert light energy into food energy.

3. The basic chemical equation for photosynthesis is:

   Carbon dioxide + Water + Light → Glucose + Oxygen

   $6\ CO_2 + 12\ H_2O + \text{Light energy} \rightarrow C_6H_{12}O_6 + 6\ O_2$

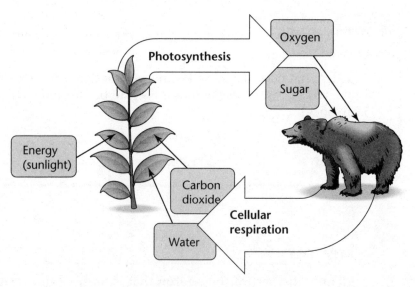

4. Organisms consume the glucose produced in photosynthesis as food to obtain energy in the process of **cellular respiration (see section 6.4).**

   Glucose + Oxygen → Carbon dioxide + Water + Energy

   $$C_6H_{12}O_6 + 6 O_2 → 6CO_2 + 12 H_2O + ATP \text{ (energy)}$$

5. Cellular respiration takes place in the mitochondria. The complex biochemical sequence known as **Krebs cycle** starts with a carbohydrate and strips it down.

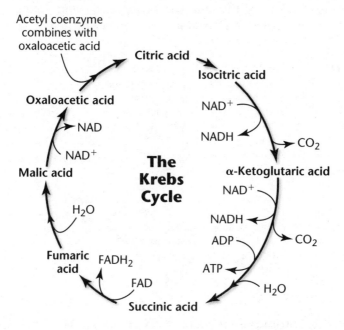

Acetyl coenzyme combines with oxaloacetic acid

Citric acid

Isocitric acid

Oxaloacetic acid

NAD^+

NAD

NADH

CO_2

NAD^+

The Krebs Cycle

α-Ketoglutaric acid

Malic acid

NAD^+

H_2O

NADH

ADP

CO_2

Fumaric acid

$FADH_2$

ATP

FAD

H_2O

Succinic acid

6. The Krebs cycle ultimately produces chemicals that are used to generate ATP, the cells' energy source.

7. Note that photosynthesis and cellular respiration are the reverse of one another.

   a. Animals consume the glucose that plants make.

   b. Plants use carbon dioxide that animals give off.

   c. Animals consume the oxygen that plants give off.

8. What do plants use for energy? The glucose that they manufacture for energy themselves! So, virtually all organisms are dependent on photosynthesis.

9. Green plants look green because the chlorophyll pigments in leaves reflect green light.

10. Chlorophyll pigments absorb low-frequency (red) and high-frequency (blue) light best, so red and blue light work best for growing plants indoors.

B. DNA and Proteins

1. **DNA** stands for deoxyribonucleic acid (a nucleic acid).

2. DNA is the hereditary material in all living things. DNA is located on chromosomes in the cell nucleus.

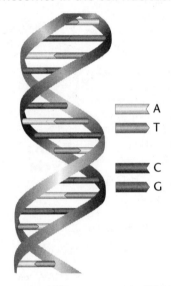

A
T

C
G

3. **Chromosomes** are primarily composed of DNA. Each gene is a section on a chromosome that codes for a **protein**.

4. DNA has a helical shape and is composed of four alphabet-like bases, A (adenine), T (thymine), C (cytosine), and G (guanine). Pairs form of A-T and C-G.

5. The sequence of bases in a **gene** code for a particular protein like letters in an alphabet.

6. To make a protein, the "alphabet" base pair code of DNA is unzipped and transcribed into **RNA**. RNA has base pairs C, G, A, and U (uracil). U replaces T (thymine) in RNA.

7. The RNA is sent out of the nucleus to the ribosomes, where proteins are made.

8. The "letters" of RNA code for **amino acids,** the building blocks of proteins.

9. Proteins as enzymes help cells carry out all of their important chemical reactions. For example, an **enzyme** helps a cell break down a sugar molecule in the mitochondria so it can be burned in a combustion reaction for energy.

10. The "central dogma" for cells is shown below. The DNA "master" code is transcribed into an RNA code. The RNA code is translated into proteins that carry out all important cell functions.

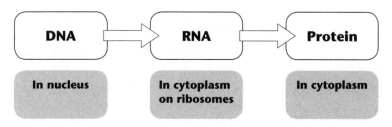

11. **Mutations** are mistakes in copying DNA. An example of mutations that cause disorders are hemophilia and Down syndrome. A single mistake such as the one shown can cause the production of a faulty protein.

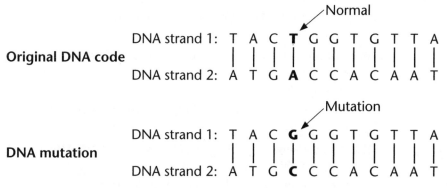

C. Mutations and Evolution

1. In 1859, Charles Darwin posed the theory of evolution, which was based on the idea of **natural selection.**

2. Natural selection states that when species change, the change can be inherited by offspring.

3. If the change proves to be advantageous, the inheritors of the trait will survive more readily than others. In this way, an organism **evolves**.

4. For example, a random change may alter the beak of a finch. (Darwin actually studied finches.) In most cases, the change will be unfavorable—such as a crooked beak—and the organism will not survive.

5. In rare cases, however, the change can be an advantage. A longer beak, for example, might allow the finch to obtain hard-to-reach food.

6. When a change is favorable and helps organisms survive, it is called an **adaptation**.

7. If the adaptation is especially favorable, the new form may out-compete others and come to dominate the population. This is how, for example, polar bears, whose ancestors presumably had dark fur, came to take over their environment.

8. What causes adaptations to occur? In 1859, Darwin didn't know. Today we know that DNA mutations (**see section 6.6 B**) cause adaptations to occur.

9. The sequence goes as follows.
   a. Random mistakes in copying DNA occur. These are mutations.
   b. Mutations produce changes in the organism that are usually harmful. For example, a bear living in the Arctic may develop extra short fur.
   c. Harmful changes, such as short fur for an Arctic bear, aren't perpetuated.
   d. Occasionally, a mutation is beneficial, such as white fur in an Arctic bear.
   e. The offspring that inherit the mutated white fur gene have an advantage over others.
   f. These white offspring thrive and have more offspring themselves. Those offspring inherit the white fur gene.
   g. Soon white-furred bears have taken over.

D. Mendelian Genetics

1. In 1865, Austrian monk Gregor Mendel crossed purebred tall (*TT*) pea plants with purebred short plants (*tt*). The result for the F$_1$ (first) generation was all tall plants.

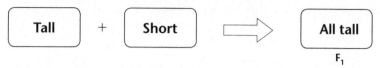

2. Mendel explained these results by suggesting that the plants had **dominant** and **recessive** genes. In the F$_1$ generation, all individuals had a dominant T (tall) gene, so they all had the tall **phenotype** (actual form).

$$\boxed{TT} \quad + \quad \boxed{tt} \quad \Longrightarrow \quad \boxed{Tt}$$
$$F_1$$

3. Crossing the F$_1$ generation with itself in a *Tt* × *Tt* pairing produces an F$_2$ generation that does have short individuals. This *Punnett square* shows the above cross.

Punnett Square F2

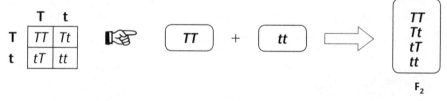

4. The **genotypes** (genetic form) and **phenotypes** (actual form) expected from this *Tt* × *Tt* cross would be $\frac{3}{4}$ tall and $\frac{1}{4}$ short.

Genotype: $\quad \frac{1}{4}\ TT + \frac{1}{4}\ Tt + \frac{1}{4}\ tT + \frac{1}{4}\ tt$

Phenotype: $\qquad\quad \frac{3}{4}$ tall $\qquad \frac{1}{4}$ short

5. For sex determination, organisms have *X* and *Y* chromosomes. An *XX* genotype creates a female; *XY* is male.

6. A sex-linked trait such as color blindness is carried only on *X* chromosomes and marked by X^C. *Y* chromosomes are "blank" for sex-linked traits—they are not expressed.

7. When a non-color-blind mother who carries the recessive color-blind X^C **allele** (X^CX) marries a normal XY father, the following genotypes result:

	X	Y
X^C	X^CX	X^CY
X	XX	XY

8. As you can see above, the female X^CX is not color blind because the X^C allele is recessive.

9. The male X^CY *is* color blind because the Y chromosome is not expressed for the color-blind gene.

6.6

Problem 1:

A scientist analyzed a sample from cells and found it to contain equal amounts of cytosine, guanine, uracil, and adenine. From which part of the cell did the sample come?

A) Ribosomes   C) Chromosomes

B) Nucleus   D) Genes

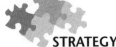 STRATEGY

Be aware of the difference between RNA and DNA.

THINK

- Cytosine, guanine, uracil, and adenine are all bases for nucleic acids. Because uracil rather than thymine is included, the sample must be RNA rather than DNA.

- RNA is located primarily on the ribosomes, not in the nucleus. Chromosomes (C) and genes (D) are both part of the nucleus (B), so they are all incorrect. This leaves (A) as the correct answer choice.

6.6

Problem 2:

A planet with plenty of carbon dioxide, water, and sunshine has no plants. How would you expect the planet to change if plants are introduced and become widespread?

A) Carbon dioxide levels will increase.

B) Oxygen levels will increase.

C) Oxygen levels will decrease.

D) Global warming will occur.

STRATEGY

Refer to the basic equation for photosynthesis.

THINK

- Photosynthesis uses water and sunlight to produce sugars and oxygen.

- As plants become widespread, they will give off oxygen to the atmosphere. This means that oxygen levels will increase, making (B) the correct response.

6.6

Problem 3:

What fraction of offspring will be short in a cross of *Tt* and *tt* parents?

A) $\frac{1}{2}$ B) $\frac{1}{4}$ C) $\frac{3}{4}$ D) All

STRATEGY

Create a Punnett square and use it find the phenotypes.

THINK

- The Punnett square shows 2 of the 4 offspring as *tt*:

	t	*t*
T	*Tt*	*Tt*
t	*tt*	*tt*

- This means that half of the offspring will be short, making (A) the correct answer choice.

6.7 ECOLOGY

A. Ecological Topics

1. An **ecosystem** consists of both **biotic** (living things, e.g., fish, bacteria, lily pads, and insects) and **abiotic** (nonliving things, e.g., air, water, and temperature) factors.

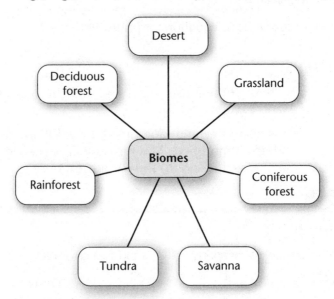

2. A **community** refers to the different organisms within an ecosystem, such as lizards, cactus, and scorpions in a desert ecosystem. **Population** refers to the number of individuals within a certain species, such as the number of collared lizards in a location. **Biomes** are very large regions that are ecologically similar.

3. Within an ecosystem, materials are continuously cycled and recycled.

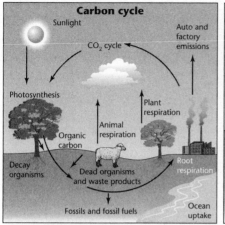

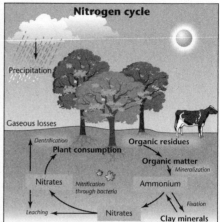

4. Organisms also constantly cycle energy. A **food web** shows relationships between **producers**, organisms such as plants that make food, and **consumers**, organisms that eat food.

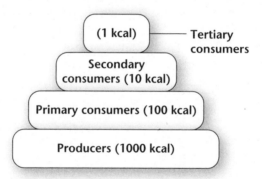

5. Energy levels in a community decrease 90% at each level. The 1000 kcal created by producers at the first level drops to 100 kcal at the primary consumer level.

6. The pattern continues until there is only 1 kcal available at the tertiary consumer (e.g., hawk and tiger) level.

7. In a food web, the arrow points *away* from the animal that is *consumed*.

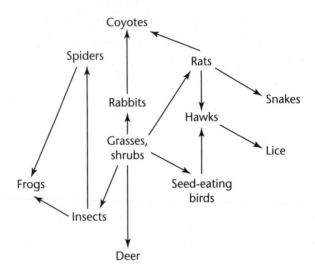

8. **Carrying capacity** refers to the size of a population that can be sustained, given the environment with respect to such things as food, water, climate, competitors, and so on.

9. If conditions are favorable, an organism's population may increase at an exponential rate until it encounters some limiting factor, such as not enough food or a devastating predator.

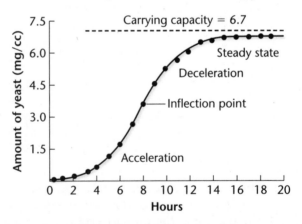

10. Organisms are identified taxonomically using the following pattern.

Category	Example	Explanation
Kingdom	Animalia	Animals
Phylum	Chordata	Backboned animals

(*continued*)

(continued)

Category	Example	Explanation
Class	*Mammal*	Mammals
Order	*Carnivora*	Meat eaters
Family	*Felidae*	Cats
Genus	*Panther*	Large cats
Species	*Tigris*	Tiger
Subspecies	*Panthera tigris tigris*	Bengal tiger

6.7

Problem 1:

Which organism is a biological producer?

A) Cow   B) Human   C) Honeybee   D) Rose bush

STRATEGY

Refer to the definition of *producer* and *consumer*.

THINK

- Although cows produce milk, humans produce many different products, and honeybees produce honey, none of them qualify as biological producers because they do not *make* food from carbon dioxide and water. This means that (A), (B), and (C) are all incorrect.

- As a plant, a rosebush carries out photosynthesis, so it is a producer, making (D) the correct response.

6.7

Problem 2:

Which organism in a food web would have arrows pointing at it but not away from it?

A) Lizard   B) Wolf   C) Grass   D) Mouse

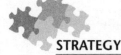

STRATEGY

Recognize how symbols in food webs are used.

THINK

- Arrows pointing at an organism indicate other life forms that are consumed by the organism.

- If arrows point only at the organism, it means that the organism consumes other life forms but is not consumed itself.

- It logically follows that the organism is a predator of some type. The wolf is the only predator that is not preyed upon, so answer choice (B) is correct.

6.7

Problem 3:

The producers in an ecosystem provide 5×10^8 kcal of energy. How much of this energy would be used by secondary consumers?

A) 5×10^{10} kcal   C) 1×10^6 kcal

B) 5×10^6 kcal   D) 0.25×10^6 kcal

STRATEGY

Refer to the relationship between producers and secondary consumers.

THINK

- Each trophic level has only 10% of the energy available from the previous level.

- Secondary consumers are two levels down from the producer level; therefore, they should have $1/10^2$ or $1/100$ energy available.

- Multiplying 5×10^8 kcal by $1/100$ gives 5×10^6 kcal, making (B) the correct answer choice.

Physical Science

EXPERIMENTAL PROCEDURE

A. Hypothesis Testing

1. Science advances largely by the use of hypothesis testing.

2. A **hypothesis** is a statement or question that can be tested.

3. Examples of hypotheses:

   - **Statement form:** Strength is proportional to the amount of training an athlete does.

   - **Question form:** Is strength proportional to athletic training?

4. To test a hypothesis, you need to conduct an **experiment**. Each group below will be tested for strength using bench press weights each week.

   - **Group 1:** 90 minutes of training per day

   - **Group 2:** 60 minutes of training per day

   - **Group 3:** 30 minutes of training per day

   - **Group 4 (Control group):** No training

5. The **independent** variable (input variable) in this experiment is the training time for each group. The **dependent** variable (output variable) is the number of pounds each group can bench press.

B. Validity and Reliability

1. A scientific procedure or experiment has **validity** if it is measuring the quantity or quality that is intended to be measured.

2. Measuring a patient's temperature is a valid way to check for infection because a raised temperature is typically associated with infections.

3. Measuring a patient's temperature is not a valid way to check for back pain because back pain does not typically result in a raised temperature.

4. A scientific procedure or experiment has **reliability** if it is repeatable over time.

5. A scale that consistently underweighs patients by 8 pounds is reliable but not valid. It consistently shows the same error, but the weight that it shows is not correct.

6. A scale sometimes registers an accurate average weight. At other times, the scale shows the weight to be too high or too low. On average, the scale is accurate. Overall this scale is somewhat valid as a measuring device but not reliable.

C. Scientific Notation

1. Scientific notation is based on powers of 10.

$$10^0 = 1$$

$$10^1 = 10 \qquad\qquad 10^{-1} = 0.1$$
$$10^2 = 100 \qquad\qquad 10^{-1} = 0.01$$
$$10^3 = 1000 \qquad\qquad 10^{-3} = 0.001$$
$$10^4 = 10,000 \qquad\qquad 10^{-4} = 0.0001$$
$$10^5 = 100,000 \qquad\qquad 10^{-5} = 0.00001$$

2. Scientific notation combines conventional numbers and numbers expressed as powers of 10.

$$3 \times 10^3 = 3 \times 1000 \qquad 5.74 \times 10^4 = 5.7 \times 10,000$$
$$= 3000 \qquad\qquad\qquad = 57,400$$

$$7 \times 10^{-1} = 7 \times 0.1 \qquad 8.297 \times 10^{-5} = 8.297 \times 0.00001$$
$$= 0.7 \qquad\qquad\qquad = 0.00008297$$

3. Scientific notation is especially good for expressing very large or very small numbers.

$$458{,}000{,}000{,}000{,}000 = 4.58 \times 10^{15}$$
$$0.000000000716 = 7.16 \times 10^{-10}$$

4. For calculation, multiply or divide the conventional numbers separately; then add or subtract the powers of 10.

$$
\begin{aligned}
4.16 \times 10^5 \times 3.1 \times 10^{-3} &= (4.16 \times 3.1) \times (10^5 \times 10^{-3}) \\
&= (12.896) \times (10^{5+\,-3}) \\
&= 12.896 \times 10^2 \\
&= 1289.6
\end{aligned}
$$

To multiply, add exponents.

$$
\begin{aligned}
20.5 \times 10^3 \div 4.1 \times 10^{-3} &= (20.5 \div 4.1) \times (10^5 \times 10^{-3}) \\
&= (5.0) \times (10^{3-\,-3}) \\
&= 5.0 \times 10^6 \\
&= 5{,}000{,}000
\end{aligned}
$$

To divide, subtract exponents.

7.1

Problem 1:

A hospital manager suspects that the pay scale for nurses and the number of complaints that the hospital receives from patients are inversely proportional. The manager is organizing a study to prove her hypothesis. Which of the following would be the dependent variable for the study?

A) Number of nurses   C) Pay scale for nurses

B) Number of complaints   D) Number of patients

STRATEGY

To find the dependent variable, identify the output item that will be measured.

THINK

- The input, or independent variable, in this study is the pay scales that are given to the nurses, making (C) incorrect.

- The output, or dependent variable, will emerge with each different level of pay, making (B) the correct answer choice.

7.1

Problem 2:

Which is greater: 0.055×10^5 or the quotient of $5 \times 10^{-1} \div 9 \times 10^{-3}$?

A) 0.055×10^5 is greater because it equals 550.

B) The quotient is greater because it equals 550.

C) The two quantities are equal.

D) The quotient is greater because it equals 55.

STRATEGY

Use the rules of scientific notation to get both quantities in the same form.

THINK

- $0.055 \times 10^5 = 5.5 \times 10^2 = 550$
- $5 \times 10^{-1} \div 9 \times 10^{-3} = (5 \div 9) \times (10^{-1 - 3})$
  $$= 0.55 \times 10^2 = 5.5 \times 10^1 = 55$$

- So the first number, equal to 550, is greater than the quotient, which equals 55, making (A) the correct response.

7.1

Problem 3:

Which of the following measurements is reliable but not valid?

A) A patient making a self-diagnosis

B) Four doctors coming up with four different diagnoses

C) Four doctors agreeing on a wrong diagnosis

D) Four doctors disagreeing about a patient's diagnosis

STRATEGY

Use the definitions for reliability and validity to draw conclusions.

THINK

- Answer choice (A) is not reliable because it is not repeatable. It is also likely not to be valid.

- Answer choice (B) is not reliable because each of the doctors came to a different conclusion.

- Answer choice (D) is not reliable because the four doctors disagree.

- Answer choice (C) is not reliable because the four doctors agree. It is not valid because the diagnosis is wrong. Therefore, (C) is the correct answer choice.

7.2 FORMS OF MATTER

A. Elements and Compounds

1. An **element** is a pure substance that cannot be broken down into different substances.

2. For example, is table salt an element? Running electricity through salt produces sodium metal and chlorine gas. Therefore, table salt is not an element.

3. Sodium and chlorine cannot be separated by any means— electrical, chemical, and so on. So sodium and chlorine are elements.

4. Elements are composed of a single kind of **atom** with a particular form, mass, and structure.

5. Atoms are composed of a central **nucleus** that contains positively charged **protons**, neutral **neutrons**, and negatively charged **electrons** that surround the nucleus.

6. Each element type has its own characteristic and **atomic number** and **atomic mass** that can be seen on the **periodic table** below.

Atomic Properties of the Elements

PERIODIC TABLE

National Institute of Standards and Technology
U.S. Department of Commerce

Physics Laboratory
physics.nist.gov

Standard Reference Data
www.nist.gov/srd

Frequently used fundamental physical constants

For the most accurate values of these and other constants, visit physics.nist.gov/constants
1 second = 9 192 631 770 periods of radiation corresponding to the transition between the two hyperfine levels of the ground state of ^{133}Cs

speed of light in vacuum	c	299 792 458 m s⁻¹	(exact)
Planck constant	h	6.6261×10^{-34} J s	($h = h/2\pi$)
elementary charge	e	1.6022×10^{-19} C	
electron mass	m_e	9.1094×10^{-31} kg	
	$m_e c^2$	0.5110 MeV	
proton mass	m_p	1.6726×10^{-27} kg	
fine-structure constant	α	1/137.036	
Rydberg constant	R_∞	10 973 732 m⁻¹	
	$R_\infty c$	$3.289 842 \times 10^{15}$ Hz	
	$R_\infty hc$	13.6057 eV	
Boltzmann constant	k	1.3807×10^{-23} J K⁻¹	

Solids
Liquids
Gases
Artificially Prepared

Atomic Number
Symbol
Name
Atomic Weight†
Ground-state Configuration
Ground-state Level
Ionization Energy (eV)

58 $^1G_4$
Ce
Cerium
140.116
[Xe]4f⁵d⁶s²
5.5387

†Based upon ^{12}C. ( ) indicates the mass number of the longest-lived isotope.

For a description of the data, visit physics.nist.gov/data

NIST SP 966 (September 2010)

7. The atomic number tells how many protons and electrons an element has. For example, sodium (abbreviated Na) has atomic number is 11, meaning that sodium has 11 protons and 11 electrons.

8. Atomic mass is computed in atomic mass units (**amu**): 1 amu for each proton and each neutron (electrons have almost no mass). Sodium's atomic mass is 11 protons +12 neutrons = 23 amu.

9. Atoms exist in different forms as **isotopes**. For example, the most common isotope of chlorine has: 17 protons + 18 neutrons = 35 amu. A rare isotope has 17 protons + 20 neutrons = 37 amu.

10. The table salt above is a pure **compound**, sodium chloride. Compounds are pure substances composed of 2 or more atoms that are bonded together.

11. On the atomic level, compounds are composed of **molecules**. Water and sugar are common compounds that are composed of molecules.

12. A water molecule is composed of hydrogen and oxygen and represented as H_2O (2 hydrogens bonded to 1 oxygen).

13. A sugar (glucose) molecule is composed of 6 carbons, 12 hydrogens, and 6 oxygens: $C_6H_{12}O_6$.

7.2

Problem 1:

How many neutrons does the element phosphorus (P) have?

A) 15   B) 16   C) 31   D) 46

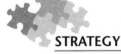

STRATEGY

Use the information on the periodic table to solve the problem.

THINK

- The number of protons (and electrons) for an element is equal to its atomic number. So phosphorus (P) has 15 protons.

- The atomic mass for P is 31.

- Atomic mass = Protons + Neutrons. So if we write an equation for n neutrons:

  $31 = 15 + n$

- Solving: $n = 16$. So phosphorus has 16 neutrons, making (B) the correct answer choice.

7.2

Problem 2:

Is hydrogen gas, H_2, an element or a compound?

A) H_2 is a compound because it has 2 atoms.

B) H_2 is an element because it has 2 atoms.

C) H_2 is an element because it has only one kind of atom.

D) H_2 is an element because it has two kinds of atoms.

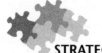

STRATEGY

Refer to the definitions of both elements and compounds.

THINK

- A compound is defined as being composed of molecules having more than one kind of atom. H_2 has only one kind of atom, hydrogen, that is bonded to itself, so H_2 cannot be a compound, meaning that (A) is incorrect.

- An element is defined as having only one kind of atom, making (C) the correct answer choice.

B. Trends in the Periodic Table

1. **Moving left to right:**

   - The **atomic radius**—distance from the nucleus to the outermost electron—decreases.
   - The **ionization energy**—energy required to remove the outermost electron—increases.
   - **Electronegativity**—attraction of an atom for electrons in a chemical bond—increases.
   - Metals and nonmetals tend to follow the trend as shown in the figure.

2. **Reason for trends in ionic radius, ionization energy, and electronegativity above:** A larger nucleus has more positive protons that keep a tighter grip on its negative electrons.

3. The outermost electrons in an atom are the **valence electrons**.

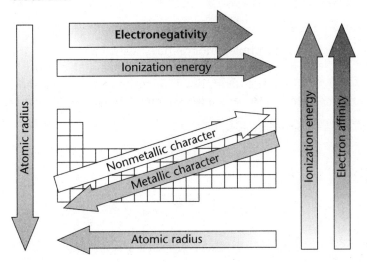

4. Atoms can lose or gain valence electrons to become **ions** with a plus or minus charge.

5. In the first few rows of the periodic table,[1] atoms "want" to fill their valence electron level with 8 electrons by either losing or gaining electrons.

---

[1]The 8 electron rule holds only for the first few rows of the periodic table, but the general principle of filling valence levels remains the same throughout the table.

6. The vertical columns in the periodic table show valence patterns, especially for the groups shown.

Column IA Alkali Metals				Column IIA Alkaline Earth Metals			
Element	Valence Electrons	Electron Loss or Gain	Ion Charge	Element	Valence Electrons	Electron Loss or Gain	Ion Charge
Li Na K	1	Lose 1 electron to have 8	+1	Be Mg Ca	2	Lose 2 electrons to have 8	+2

Column VIA Non-Metals				Column IIA Halogens			
Element	Valence Electrons	Electron Loss or Gain	Ion Charge	Element	Valence Electrons	Electron Loss or Gain	Ion Charge
O S	6	Gain 2 electrons to have 8	−2	F Cl Br	7	Gain 1 electron to have 8	−1

7. For example, fluorine has 7 valence electrons. It tends to pick up 1 electron to make 8 and have a −1 charge. Sodium, on the other hand, has 1 valence electron, so it tends to lose that 1 to have a full valence amount of 8 in its previous level.

C. Chemical Bonds

👉 Ionic bond

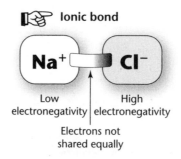

Low electronegativity | High electronegativity

Electrons not shared equally

👉 Covalent bond

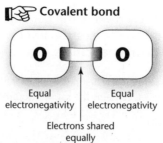

Equal electronegativity | Equal electronegativity

Electrons shared equally

1. Atoms that differ greatly in electronegativity such as Na and Cl join to form an **ionic bond**. Na gets rid of an electron to become an Na^{+1} ion. Cl gains an electron to become a Cl^- ion.

2. In an ionic bond, the atom higher in electronegativity "owns" the electrons to allow both atoms to have their valence levels filled.

3. Because electronegativity is low on the left side of the periodic table (see section 7.2 B) and high on the right side, atoms from opposite sides of the table such as halogens and alkali metals form ionic bonds:

   Ionic bonds: Na^+—Cl^-, K^+—Br^-, Ca^{2+}—$2\ F^-$, Mg^{2+}—O^{2-}

4. **Covalent bonds** form between atoms with similar or identical electronegativity:

   Covalent bonds: N_2, CO_2, H_2, CCl_4, NO_2

5. In a covalent bond, electrons are shared to fill the valence level of both atoms with 8 electrons.

7.2

Problem 3:

Which element has the smallest ionic radius?

A) Sulfur   C) Magnesium

B) Phosphorus   D) Sodium

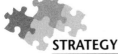

STRATEGY

Follow the trend in the periodic table for atomic radius.

THINK

- Atomic radius decreases from left to right on the periodic table.

- The element farthest to the right has the smallest atomic radius. Sulfur is furthest right, so it is the correct response.

7.2

Problem 4:

Which two elements would be most likely to form an ionic bond?

A) Carbon and nitrogen

B) Iodine and carbon

C) Sodium and iodine

D) Two atoms of bromine

STRATEGY

Find the two elements that differ the most in electronegativity.

THINK

- Electronegativity is greatest on the right side of the periodic table and lowest on the left side.

- Ionic bonds form between one element high in electronegativity and one element that is low.

- Iodine and sodium make up the only pair that includes elements from opposite sides of the periodic table, so answer choice (C) is correct.

7.3 CHEMICAL REACTIONS

A. Energy of Reaction

1. A chemical reaction occurs when chemical bonds are broken and new bonds form.

2. In a chemical reaction, matter is never created or destroyed. This concept is referred to as the law of conservation of matter.

3. For example, when a log is burned (combustion), if you carefully weigh the log before and the ash plus gases that escape afterward, you will find that they are equal.

4. **Endothermic** reactions will not occur without energy being supplied. *Endothermic* means to absorb heat.

5. Photosynthesis is an example of an endothermic reaction. Light energy is required to carry out the reaction.

$$6 \ CO_2 + 12 \ H_2O + \text{Light energy} \rightarrow C_6H_{12}O_6 + 6 \ O_2$$

6. **Exothermic** reactions are spontaneous and do not require energy to be supplied. *Exothermic* means to give off heat.

7. When sodium and chlorine are put together, they react exothermically to give off energy.

$$2 \ Na + Cl_2 \rightarrow NaCl + \text{Energy}$$

7.3

Problem 1:

Which statement is true of the photosynthesis reaction?

$$6 \ CO_2 + 12 \ H_2O + \text{Light energy} \rightarrow C_6H_{12}O_6 + 6 \ O_2$$

A) It is exothermic.

B) The carbon dioxide and sugar molecules are equal in weight.

C) As an endothermic reaction, the sum of sugar and oxygen is greater in mass than the sum of carbon dioxide and water.

D) The sum of the products, sugar and oxygen, is equal in mass to the sum of the reactants, carbon dioxide and water.

STRATEGY

Refer to the law of conservation of mass.

THINK

- Mass is never created or destroyed.

- In a reaction, the reactants (what you start with) always need to be equal in mass to the products (what you end up with).

- In this reaction, matter is conserved. That makes (D) the correct answer choice.

B. Reaction Types

1. There are four basic types of reaction, synthesis, decomposition, single replacement, and double replacement.

2. In a **synthesis** reaction, two or more elements or compounds come together to form a single compound.

Synthesis	
Pattern	**Examples**
$A + B \rightarrow AB$	$C + O_2 \rightarrow CO_2$ $3\ H_2 + N_2 \rightarrow 2\ NH_3$

3. In a **decomposition** reaction, a single compound decomposes into two or more elements or compounds.

Decomposition	
Pattern	**Examples**
$AB \rightarrow A + B$	$2\ H_2O_2 \rightarrow 2\ H_2O + O_2$ $ZnCl_2 \rightarrow Zn + Cl_2$

4. In a **single replacement** reaction, one element switches places and replaces another element. Note that Cu and Ag switch places in the reaction below.

Single Replacement	
Pattern	**Example**
$AB + C \rightarrow AC + B$	$Cu + 2\ AgNO_3 \rightarrow Cu(NO_3)_2 + 2\ Ag$

5. In a **double replacement** reaction, two elements switch places and replace one another. Note that NO_3 and Cl switch places in the reaction below.

Double Replacement	
Pattern	**Example**
$AB + CD \rightarrow AD + CB$	$AgNO_3 + NaCl \rightarrow AgCl + NaNO_3$

7.2

Problem 2:

What kind of reaction is $2\,Al + Fe_2O_3 \rightarrow Al_2O_3 + 2Fe$?

A) Decomposition

B) Double displacement

C) Single displacement

D) Synthesis

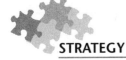

STRATEGY

Compare the reaction with the models above.

THINK

- In this reaction, the Al atoms replace the Fe atoms to form an oxide, so it is clearly a displacement, meaning that answer choices (A) and (D) are incorrect.

- If this were double displacement, two compounds would "trade" partners. Because only one compound changes, this is a single displacement, making answer choice (C) correct.

C. Balanced Equations

1. All chemical equations must be balanced—that is, the atoms on the left side of the equation must be accounted for on the right side.

2. You can check to see whether the single replacement reaction above is balanced.

$$Cu + 2\,AgNO_3 \rightarrow Cu(NO_3)_2 + 2\,Ag$$

3. Make a table to compare of all atoms on the left side with all of the atoms on the right side.

4. The table shows that the equation is balanced.

Left Side			
Cu	2 AgNO$_3$		
Cu	Ag	N	O
1 × 1	2 × 1	2 × 1	2 × 3
1	2	2	6

Right Side			
2 Ag	Cu(NO$_3$)$_2$		
Ag	Cu	N	O
2 × 1	1 × 1	2 × 1	2 × 3
2	1	2	6

7.3

Problem 3:

Which of the following shows a balanced equation?

A) $C_3H_8 + 5 O_2 \rightarrow 2 CO_2 + H_2O$

B) $C_3H_8 + 3 O_2 \rightarrow 2 CO_2 + 3 H_2O$

C) $2 C_3H_8 + 5 O_2 \rightarrow 3 CO_2 + 4 H_2O$

D) $C_3H_8 + 5 O_2 \rightarrow 3 CO_2 + 4 H_2O$

STRATEGY

Make a table to compare atoms on each side of the equation.

THINK

• Make a table.

Left Side		
C$_3$H$_8$		5 O$_2$
C	H	O
3 × 1	8 × 1	5 × 2
3	8	10

Right Side			
3 CO$_2$		4 H$_2$O	
C	O	H	O
3 × 1	3 × 2	4 × 2	4 × 1
3	6	8	4

- There are 3 carbons on each side and 8 hydrogens.
- From the table, you can see that the left and right sides match up if you add 6 Os to 4 Os to obtain 10 Os.

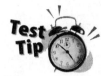

You can rule out answer choices simply by looking at a single atom. The left side has 3 carbons and the right only 2, so (A) and (B) are both incorrect. For (C), the left side has 6 carbons and the right only 3, so it also can be ruled out.

7.4 PHASES OF MATTER

A. Phases

1. Atoms and molecules of the same type have a natural attraction to one another.

2. Depending on temperature and (air) pressure, every form of matter can exist in three different phases—**solid, liquid,** and **gas.**

3. In the graph above, water is heated to boiling.

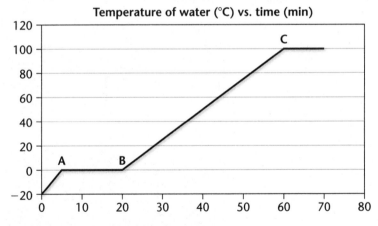

4. Heat increases the KE (see section 9.8 C) of the water molecules and speeds them up. Raising the temperature to 0°C turns ice to liquid (A).

5. While heating, the icy water will remain at 0° until it completely turns to liquid (B).

6. Water temperature will continue to rise until it reaches 100°C, at which point it will boil (C). The water will remain at 100° until it completely turns to gas.

7. Phase changes can require heat (endothermic) or give off heat (exothermic).

Phase	Change	Energy
Solid to liquid	Melting	Endothermic
Liquid to gas	Vaporizing	Endothermic
Gas to liquid	Condensing	Exothermic
Liquid to solid	Freezing	Exothermic
Solid to gas	Sublimation	Endothermic
Gas to solid	Deposition	Exothermic

8. All forms of matter change state in a similar way. Wood alcohol, for example, boils at 64.7°C rather than 100°C like water. Wood alcohol won't freeze until the temperature reaches −97.8°C.

9. Changing the air pressure will change melting and boiling temperatures. For example, increasing the pressure will cause most substances to melt and boil at a temperature that is higher than normal.[2]

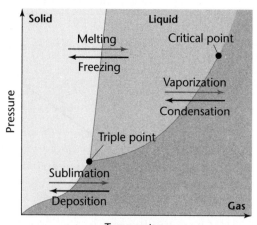

[2]Water is unusual in that increasing pressure causes it to melt at a temperature that is lower than normal. This is because squeezing water with pressure breaks up its crystal-like structure.

B. Density and Buoyancy

 1. **Density** is the amount of mass a substance has per unit volume.

 2. Density is measured in units of mass or weight per volume (e.g., g/cm^3). (Note: $1\ cm^3 = 1\ ml$, so the units of milliliters and cubic centimeters can be interchanged freely.)

 3. A $4\ cm^3$ (cubic centimeter, also cc) rock that weighs 60 g and has a density of:

    $60\ g \div 4\ cm^3 = 15\ g/cm^3$

 4. Water has a density of $1\ g/1\ ml$. Items with a density greater than water sink in liquid water; items with a lower density float.

 5. For example, the rock above has a density of 15 g/ml, so its density is greater than that of water. Therefore, it will sink.

7.4

Problem 1:

A liquid boils at 50°C. Which of the following will most likely happen if the air pressure is lowered?

A) The liquid will boil at 55°C.

B) The liquid will boil at 45°C.

C) The liquid will freeze at a higher temperature than normal.

D) The liquid will condense at a higher temperature than normal.

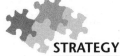

STRATEGY

Decreasing pressure puts less of a "squeeze" on the substance, making it easier to boil.

THINK

- Pressure squeezes matter together.

- Squeezing a gas forces particles to be closer together and therefore makes it harder to boil, raising the boiling temperature.

- Conversely, lowering the pressure makes it easier to boil the liquid, lowering the boiling temperature, making (B) the correct response.

- Note that a lower pressure will keep particles apart and prevent them from freezing, making (C) incorrect.

- Similarly, (D) is incorrect because lower pressure will make it harder for the liquid to condense, lowering the temperature of condensation.

7.4

Problem 2:

A 20 ml of olive oil weighs 18.36 g. Will an 8-g chunk of plastic that has a volume of 11 cm^3 float in olive oil?

A) Yes, because the plastic's density is greater than that of the oil.

B) Yes, because the plastic's density is less than that of the oil.

C) No, because the plastic's density is 0.73 g/cm^3.

D) No, because the oil's density is 0.92 g/cm^3.

STRATEGY

Calculate the density of both items. If the plastic has a lower density, it will float.

THINK

- Olive oil density = Weight/Volume = 18.36/20 = 0.92 g/cm^3.

- Plastic density = Weight/Volume = 8/1 = 0.73 g/cm^3.

- The density of plastic is less so it will float, making (B) the correct answer choice.

7.5 PROPORTIONALITY AND GAS LAWS

A. Proportionality

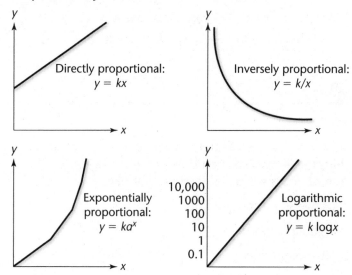

Directly proportional:
$y = kx$

Inversely proportional:
$y = k/x$

Exponentially proportional:
$y = ka^x$

10,000
1000
100
10
1
0.1

Logarithmic proportional:
$y = k \log x$

1. Direct proportionality has the form $y = kx$, where k is a constant. Any straight line graph is likely to exhibit direct proportionality where:

   • Increase in $x \rightarrow$ Increase in y
   • Decrease in $x \rightarrow$ Decrease in y

2. Inverse proportionality has the form $y = k/x$, where k is a constant. Any graph showing a hyperbole shape is likely to exhibit inverse proportionality where:

   • Increase in $x \rightarrow$ Decrease in y
   • Decrease in $x \rightarrow$ Increase in y

3. Exponential proportionality has the form $y = ka^x$, where a and k constants. Any parabola-shaped graph is likely to exhibit exponential proportionality where:

   • Increase in $x \rightarrow$ Large increase in y
   • Decrease in $x \rightarrow$ Large decrease in y

4. Logarithmic proportionality has the form $y = k \log x$ and appears as a straight line on a logarithmic scale that increases by a power of 10 every interval:

- Increase in $x \rightarrow$ Large increase in y
- Decrease in $x \rightarrow$ Large decrease in y

7.5

Problem 1:

Data show that the greater number of hours that nurses work on a shift, the less satisfaction they get from their job. What would a graph of hours versus satisfaction look like?

A) Positive slope straight line

B) Parabola upward

C) Flat straight line

D) Downward hyperbola

STRATEGY

Match the situation to the type of proportionality.

THINK

- As hours increase, satisfaction decreases. This is clearly an inverse relationship.
- A graph of an inverse relationship is downward and hyperbolic in shape, making (D) the correct response.

B. Gas Laws

1. Charles' law states that temperature and volume are directly proportional.

$$\frac{V_1}{T_1} = \frac{V_2}{T_2}$$

2. The gas laws are carried out in the Kelvin temperature scale in which 0° equals −273°C.

Charles' law

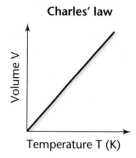

Temperature T (K)

7.5

Problem 2:

An expandable container has a volume of 1000 ml at a temperature of 27°C. The temperature is raised to 47°C. What is the new volume of the container?

A) 1740.7 ml   C) 1066.7 ml

B) 2000 ml   D) 2000 ml

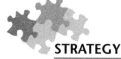

STRATEGY

Apply Charles' law using temperatures in Kelvin.

THINK

- Kelvin degrees = Celsius degrees + 273°
- Applying the equation above, we get:
- T_1 = 27°C + 273°C = 300°K
- T_2 = 47°C + 273°C = 320°K
- Now substitute for $V_1/T_1 = V_2/T_2$:
- 1000/300 = V_2/320
- Solving, V_2 = 1066.7 ml, making (C) the correct response.

3. Boyle's law states that pressure and volume are inversely proportional.

$$P_1V_1 = P_2V_2$$

Boyle's law

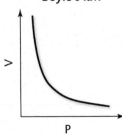

7.5

Problem 3:

An expandable container has a volume of 1500 ml at a pressure of 750 torr. The pressure is raised to 800 torr. By how much does the volume change?

A) 100 ml   B) 1600 ml   C) 1400 ml   D) 1066.7 ml

STRATEGY

Apply Boyle's law using temperatures in Kelvin.

THINK

- Substitute for $P_1V_1 = P_2V_2$:
- $(1500)(750) = V_2(800)$
- Solving, $V_2 = 1600$ ml
- That is an increase of 1500 ml + n = 1600 ml.
- Solving for n: $n = 100$ ml, making (A) the correct response.

7.6 SOLUTIONS

A. Physical Changes, Chemical Changes, and Mixtures

1. Physical properties include such qualities as shape, color, texture, size, boiling point, and so on.

2. **Physical changes** do not require a change in chemical composition. Water undergoes a physical change when it freezes or melts. Both liquid water and ice have the chemical composition H_2O.

3. **Chemical changes** require a change in chemical composition. New molecules are formed. Methane, CH_4, undergoes a chemical change during combustion. CH_4 turns into carbon dioxide and water.

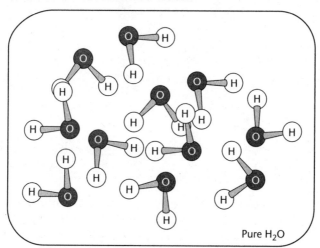

Pure H_2O

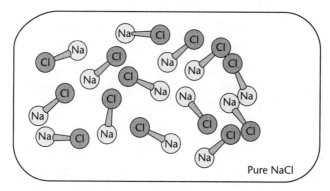

Pure NaCl

$$CH_4 + 2\,O_2 \rightarrow CO_2 + 2\,H_2O$$

4. As you know from section 7.2 A, elements and compounds are pure substances. Elements cannot be broken down by any conventional means.

5. Compounds can be broken down only by chemical changes (reactions) that break chemical bonds.

6. All particles in an element or compound are identical. Water is composed of trillions of identical H_2O molecules. Sodium chloride is composed of trillions of NaCl particles.

7. Particles in a **mixture** are not identical. A **heterogeneous** mixture is not uniform. A salad or beach sand is an example of a heterogeneous mixture.

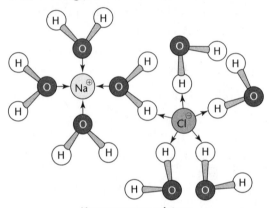

Homogeneous mixture

8. A homogeneous mixture is uniform. A **solution** is an example of a homogeneous mixture. The substance dissolved in a solution is the **solute**. The dissolving substance is the **solvent**.

9. NaCl dissolves in water as ions and forms a solution. These ions become surrounded by water molecules.

10. A homogeneous solution such as sugar water or air is clear and transparent. A heterogenous mixture such as milk or muddy water is not clear.

11. Solutions can take on many forms. Air is a solution. So is steel, which is an alloy of iron, carbon, and other elements.

Solutions		
Solvent	**Solute**	**Example**
Liquid	Liquid	Alcohol in water
Liquid	Solid	Sugar in water
Liquid	Gas	Oxygen in water
Gas	Gas	Nitrogen in air
Gas	Solid	Soot in air
Solid	Solid	Metal–metal alloy

7.6

Problem 1:

The figure shows which of the following?

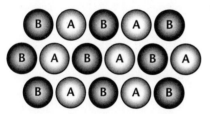

A) Heterogeneous mixture, possibly a solution

B) Homogeneous mixture, possibly a solution

C) Heterogeneous mixture, not a solution

D) An element, not a solution

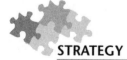

STRATEGY

Refer to the discussion of mixtures and solutions.

THINK

- The group is clearly not an element or compound because it is composed of different particles, making (D) incorrect.

- A heterogenous mixture is not uniform or orderly, so (A) is incorrect. Also, a solution must be homogeneous, not heterogeneous.

- This mixture is homogeneous and could be a solution, making (B) the correct response. If visually it appears clear, then it would be likely to be categorized as a solution.

B. Solubility and Concentration

1. The **solubility**, or ability to dissolve, depends on the solvent and solute.

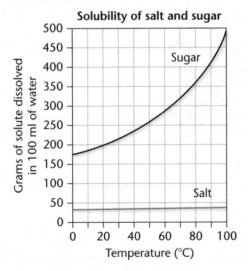

Solubility of salt and sugar

2. The graph shows that solubility for sugar (glucose) increases significantly with temperature. Salt only increases very slightly as temperatures rise.

3. **Concentration**, the amount of solute dissolved per liter, can be computed by finding the ratio of solute to solvent.

7.6

Problem 2:

45 grams of NaCl is dissolved in an 80-ml solution. What is the concentration of NaCl?

A) 37.5%   C) 56.25%

B) 45%   D) 48.8%

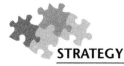

STRATEGY

Find the percentage of NaCl in the entire solution.

THINK

- 45 out of 80 = 45/80
- 45/80 = 0.5625 = 56.25%
- This makes (C) the correct response.

C. Moles

1. Atoms are incredibly tiny. Each hydrogen atom weighs 0.00000000000000000000000166 g or 1.66×10^{-24} g.

2. To deal with practical numbers, chemists invented the **mole**, a number equal to 6.023×10^{23}.

   > A mole is simply the name for a number in the same way that a dozen is a name for 12. A mole is a name for 6.023×10^{23}.

3. One mole of hydrogen atoms has a mass of 1 g. One mole of carbon atoms has a mass of 12 g.

4. Moles are set up to match amu numbers on the periodic table. Note that you can have a mole of a compound, such as CO_2 and O_2, as well as a mole of an element.

Element	Mass of 1 Atom (atomic mass)	Mass of 1 Mole, 6.023×10^{23} Particles (molar mass)
H	1 amu	1 g
C	12 amu	12 g
O	16 amu	16 g
Cl	35.5 amu	35.5 g
Au	197 amu	197 g
CO_2	44 amu	44 g
O_2	32 amu	32 g

5. Molecular/molar mass or molar mass can be found on the periodic table. To find the molecular/molar mass of CCl_4:

- $CCl_4 = 1 \text{ C} + 4 \text{ Cl}$
  $= (12 \text{ amu}) + (4 \times 35.5 \text{ amu})$
  $= 286 \text{ amu/molecule or } 286 \text{ g/mole}$

6. You can find a fraction of a mole just like you can find the fraction of a number. For carbon in grams:

- $\quad$ 1 mole = 12 g
  $\quad$ 0.5 mole = (0.5)(12 g/mole)
  $\qquad\quad = 6 \text{ g}$

For carbon in atoms:

- 1 mole = 6.02×10^{23} particles (atoms or molecules)
- 0.5 mole = $(0.5)(6.02 \times 10^{23}$ atoms/mole)
  $\qquad\qquad = 3.01 \times 10^{23}$ particles

7.6

Problem 3:

What is the molar weight of glucose $C_6H_{12}O_6$?

A) 120 g   C) 180 amu

B) 40 amu   D) 180 g

STRATEGY

Add up the molar mass of each element separately.

THINK

- Molar mass is expressed in grams.
- $C_6H_{12}O_6 = 6\,C + 12\,H + 6\,O$
  $= (6 \times 12\ g) + (12 \times 1\ g) + (6 \times 16\ g)$
  $= 180\ g$
- This makes (D) the correct response.

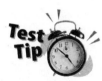

Test Tip

Note that (B) and (C) are expressed in amu, not grams, so they are incorrect answer choices.

7.6

Problem 4:

How many molecules are in 2.25 moles of CO_2?

A) 1.35×10^{23} C) 13.45 g

B) 1.35×10^{24} D) 3.7×10^{22}

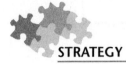

Use a proportion to solve.

THINK

- If 1 mole has 6.02×10^{23} molecules, then you can write a proportion.

- 1 mole/6.02×10^{23} molecules = 2.25 moles/n molecules.

- Solving for n: $n = 13.45 \times 10^{23}$. Moving the decimal point 1 place over gives 1.35×10^{24} molecules, making (B) the correct response.

- Note that (C) must be incorrect because it is expressed in grams.

D. Molarity

1. The concentration of a solution can be expressed in grams per liter (see section 7.6B) or as molarity.

2. **Molarity** is expressed in moles per liter (M) of solution. A 1-M solution of NaCl contains exactly 1 mole of NaCl in exactly 1 liter of solution.

3. Example: A nurse dissolved 80 g of HCl (hydrochloric acid) in a 60-ml solution. What was the molarity of the solution?

   a. Find molar mass of HCl = (1 H) + 1 Cl
   $$= 1 + 35.5 = 36.5 \text{ g/mol}$$

   b. Write a proportion to find moles of HCl:

   80 g HCl/n mol = 36.5 g/1 mol
   $$n = 2.2 \text{ mol HCl}$$

   c. Find moles per liter of solution:

   2.2 mol / 0.6 l = 3.67 M

4. Example: How many grams of NH_3 are in 1.5 l of a 0.8 M solution?

   a. Find molar mass of $NH_3 = (1\ N) + (3\ H)$
$$= 18\ g/mol$$

   b. Write a proportion to find moles of NH_3:

       $0.8\ mol\ NH_3/1\ l = n\ mol\ NH_3/1.5\ l$
$$n = 1.2\ mol\ NH_3$$

   c. Find the number of grams of NH_3:

       $(1.2\ mol) \times 18\ g/mol = 21.6\ g\ NH_3$

7.6

Problem 5:

What is the molarity of the solution in which 400 g of sucrose, $C_{11}H_{22}O_{11}$, is dissolved in water to make a 350-ml solution?

A) 3.34 M   C) 6.68 M

B) 0.334 M   D) 1.67 M

STRATEGY

Find the number of moles of sucrose that you have. Then use that number to find molarity.

THINK

- Find the number of moles of sucrose that has a mass of 400 grams.

- $C_{11}H_{22}O_{11} = 11\ C + 22\ H + 11\ O$
$$= (11 \times 12\ g) + (22 \times 1\ g) + (11 \times 16\ g)$$
$$= 342\ g/mol$$

- Write a proportion to find moles of $C_{11}H_{22}O_{11}$:

  400 g $C_{11}H_{22}O_{11}/n$ mol = 342 g/1 mol

  n = 1.17 mol $C_{11}H_{22}O_{11}$

- Find moles per liter of solution:

  1.17 mol / 0.35 l = 3.34 M

- This makes (A) the correct response.

E. Acids and Bases

   1. **Acids** are compounds that:

     a. Ionize in water

     b. Have a sour taste

     c. Turn litmus paper red

     d. Have a pH less than 7.0

     e. React readily with bases and many metals

     f. Donate H^+ ions in solution

   2. **Bases** are compounds that:

     a. Ionize in water

     b. Have a bitter taste

     c. Turn litmus paper blue

     d. Have a pH greater than 7.0

     e. React readily with acids

     f. Donate OH^- ions in solution

   3. The **pH** scale measures acidity from 0 (strong acid) to 14 (strong base). Water has a pH of 7.0 and is neutral.

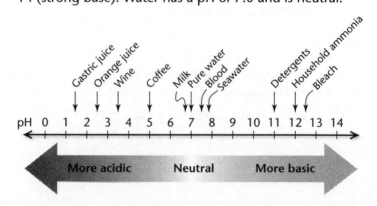

4. The pH scale has a log scale. A pH of 6.0 is 10 times as acidic as a pH of 7.0. A pH of 5.0 is 100 times as acidic as a pH of 7.0. Similarly, a pH of 9.0 is 100 times more basic than a pH of 7.0.

5. **Litmus paper** is another way to measure pH. When dipped, an acidic solution turns litmus paper red, and a base turns it blue.

6. Common acids include HCl (hydrochloric acid), vinegar, HNO_3 (nitric acid), and H_2SO_4 (sulfuric acid). Common bases include NaOH (sodium hydroxide) and $NaHCO_3$ (sodium bicarbonate).

7. Acid–base reactions occur readily. When strong acid HCl (pH 1.0) reacts with a strong base NaOH (pH 13.0), it produces a salt (NaCl) and neutral water. Acids also react strongly with some metals to produce H_2 gas.

$HCl + NaOH \rightarrow NaCl + H_2O$ (Acid–base neutralization)

$HCl + Zn \rightarrow ZnCl + H_2$ (Acid + Metal $\rightarrow H_2$)

7.6

Problem 6:

Lemon juice is about 1000 times more acidic than coffee, which has a pH of 5. What is the pH of lemon juice?

A) 1.0   C) 4.0

B) 2.0   D) 9.0

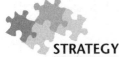

STRATEGY

Count by powers of 10 on the pH scale.

THINK

- Each unit on the logarithmic pH scale is 10 times more acidic than the previous unit.

- $1000 = 10^3$, so count three units back from pH 5.

- pH 5 – 3 units = pH 2. So answer choice (B) is the correct response.

7.7 MOTION

A. Displacement, Speed, and Velocity

1. **Displacement** is the distance an object moves when it changes position. For example, suppose bicycle rider 1 travels 100 m east in 10 seconds.

> **Velocity** and **displacement** are vector quantities that include a value *and* a direction. **Speed** and **distance** are the nonvector versions of these measurements.

   Displacement = 100 m east

   Time = 10 s

2. **Velocity** measures the speed and direction of a moving object. You can compute velocity (or average speed) by dividing distance by time.

   Average velocity = Change in displacement/Change in time

   $$= \Delta y / \Delta x = 100 / 10 \text{ s}$$

   $$= 10 \text{ m/s}$$

3. On the distance versus time graph, a straight line means that the object is moving at a constant speed.

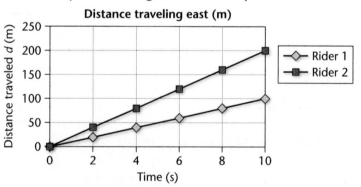

Distance traveling east (m)

4. The **slope** of the line indicates the magnitude of the speed. Thus, rider 2 is moving at a faster speed than rider 1.

5. If the graph shows a nonstraight line, the object is not moving at a constant speed.

7.7

Problem 1:

In the distance versus time graph above, what is the average speed of rider 2?

A) 10 m/s   C) 20 mph

B) 20 m/s   D) 200 m/s

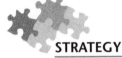

STRATEGY

Use any two points on the graph to compute the average speed.

THINK

- To find the slope, calculate $\Delta y / \Delta x$ = for any two points on the graph.
- Choose points (2,40) and (6,120).
- $\Delta y / \Delta x = 120 - 40 / 6 - 2 = 80/4 = 20$.
- So the speed is 20 m/s, making (B) the correct answer choice.

B. Acceleration

1. A straight line distance versus time graph shows constant speed. A nonstraight line graph shows an object that is changing speed.

2. Rider 3's **instantaneous speed** from time $t = 0$ to $t = 2$ is 0 — the rider is not moving. From $t = 2$ to $t = 3$, rider 3 is moving at a constant speed; then he stops from $t = 3$ to $t = 4$.

3. Rider 4's average instantaneous speed changes each second:

Speed 0−1 s $= \Delta y/\Delta x = 10 - 0 / 1 - 0 = 10/1$

  $= 10$ m/s

Speed 1−2 s $= \Delta y/\Delta x = 30 - 10 / 1 - 0 = 20/1$

  $= 20$ m/s

Speed 2−3 s $= \Delta y/\Delta x = 60 - 30 / 1 - 0 = 30/1$

  $= 30$ m/s

Speed 3−4 s $= \Delta y/\Delta x = 100 - 60 / 1 - 0 = 40/1$

  $= 40$ m/s

4. Velocity changing over time is **acceleration**. Positive acceleration is speeding up. Negative acceleration is slowing down. Units of acceleration are distance per second squared (e.g., m/s^2).

Acceleration = Δ Velocity/Δ Time

Time (s)	Velocity (m/s)
0	0
1	10
2	20
3	30
4	40
5	50

5. The data table shows **constant acceleration** of 10 m/s^2. In other words, the object's velocity is increasing by 10 m/s each second.

7.7

Problem 2:

An object accelerates at a constant rate of 5.4 m/s². How long will it take to reach a speed of 24 m/s?

A) 129.6 s   C) 4.44 s

B) 29.4 s   D) 18.6 s

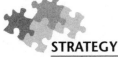

STRATEGY

Use the concept of constant acceleration to write an equation.

THINK

- Constant acceleration of 5.4 m/s² means that the object's speed increases by 5.4 m/s every second.

- $v_{final} = 24 = $ acceleration $\times t$

- $24 = (5.4)t$

- Solving for t, you get 4.44 seconds, making (C) the correct answer choice.

C. Gravity

1. A special type of acceleration is the force of **gravity**. Gravity attracts all objects toward one another. The force of gravity is weak and proportional to mass, so it is negligibly small except when one of the objects, such as the Earth, is extremely massive.

2. A free-falling object shows the force of gravity to be 9.8 m/s². The table shows the speed of a falling object.

t	0	1	2	3	4	5
Speed	0	9.8	19.6	29.4	39.2	49.0

3. How far does a free-falling object fall? To compute d, displacement, use the formula for objects with constant acceleration:

$$d = t(v_{final} - v_{initial})/2$$

7.7

Problem 3:

A 10-kg object and a 5-kg object are both dropped from a tall building. How far will they each travel after 4 seconds?

A) They each fall 78.4 m.

B) They each fall 49.2 m.

C) The 10-kg object falls 78.4 m, and the 5-kg object falls 39.2 m.

D) The 10-kg object falls 78.4 m, and the 5-kg object falls 39.2 m.

STRATEGY

Use the formula for computing distance.

THINK

- Gravity is a force that imposes constant acceleration on objects, so the formula $d = t(v_f - v_i)/2$ can be used.

$$d = t(v_f - v_i)/2$$
$$= 4(4(9.8) - 0)/2$$
$$= 4(39.2)/2$$
$$= 78.4 \text{ m}$$

- Note that the formula works for *all* falling objects regardless of their mass. So the 10-kg and 5-kg objects fall at the exact same rate. This makes (A) the correct response.

Test Tip

You can eliminate choices (C) and (D) immediately if you recognize that the 10-kg and 5-kg object both fall at the same rate.

D. Newton's Laws and Force

1. **Newton's first law** states that all objects have **inertia** that causes them to stay in motion at the same speed in the same direction unless they are acted on by an unbalanced force.

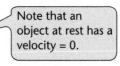

Note that an object at rest has a velocity = 0.

2. A **force** is something that causes an object to accelerate. Forces can come from pushes, pulls, friction, electrical force, and gravity.

3. In **Newton's second law**, the equation $F = ma$ identifies force on any object, where m is mass and a is acceleration. The units of force are newtons (N). $1\ N = 1\ kg \bullet 1\ m/s^2$.

4. For example, a force of 1 N will set an object in motion with an acceleration of 1 m/s^2.

$$F = ma$$

$$= (1\ kg)(1\ m/s^2) = 1\ N$$

5. If an object is at rest (velocity = 0) then:

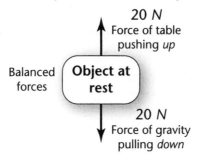

20 N
Force of table pushing *up*

Balanced forces

Object at rest

20 N
Force of gravity pulling *down*

a. Mo forces are acting on it or

b. The forces acting on it are balanced.

c. Newton's first law states that the object will stay at rest unless a force acts on it.

6. If an object is accelerating:

a. It is currently being acted on by an unbalanced force.

7. If an object is moving at a constant velocity:

    a. An unbalanced force caused it to move originally.

    b. Newton's first law says that it will stay moving at the same velocity unless acted on by a new force.

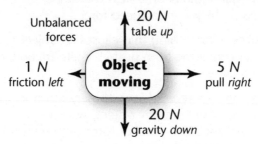

8. Newton's **third law** states that forces come in pairs. For every action there is a corresponding reaction. When you push against a wall with a force of 100 *N*, the wall pushes back at you in the opposite direction with an equal force, 100 *N*.

7.7

Problem 4:

A constant force of 18 *N* is applied to a 3-kg rock for 4 seconds. What speed will the rock reach (assume no friction)?

A) 54 m/s B) 12 m/s C) 6 m/s D) 24 m/s

STRATEGY

Use the equation $F = ma$ for $t = 4$ seconds.

THINK

- The force applied is 18 *N*. The mass of the rock is 3 kg.

- $F = ma$
  $18\ N = (3\ kg)a$
  $a = 6\ m/s^2$

- The force was applied for 4 seconds. So the rock will increase in speed by 6 m/s each second:
- 4 seconds $\times$ 6 m/s^2 = 24 m/s
- This makes (D) the correct response.

E. Gravitational Force

1. The gravitational force, g, on Earth for any object is given as:
   g = 9.8 N / kg

2. The force of gravity on a 10-kg object is:
   $$F_{gravity} = \text{Mass} \times g \text{ (gravitational force)}$$
   $$= 10 \text{ kg } (9.8 \text{ N / kg})$$
   $$= 98 \text{ N}$$

3. The 10-kg object above also applies a force to Earth. Why don't you see the Earth move?

   a. Because $F = ma$, the acceleration of an object is proportional to its mass.

   b. Compare equations for each object. The force on each object is the same. But Earth has a mass of 6 $\times$ 10^{24} kg:

   $$F_{10kg} = F_{Earth}$$
   $$m_{10kg} \bullet a_{10kg} = m_{Earth} \bullet a_{Earth}$$
   $$10 \text{ kg} \bullet a_{10kg} = 6{,}000{,}000{,}000{,}000{,}000{,}000{,}000{,}000 \bullet a_{Earth}$$

   c. As you can see, the value of a_{Earth} is incredibly tiny. But Earth does accelerate a very small amount in response to a 10-kg object.

4. Other planets are larger or smaller than Earth, so they have different values for g. On a smaller planet such as Mercury, the gravitational force is only 0.38 g. On a large planet like Jupiter, g is 2.6 g.

   Your **weight** will change depending on your planet.

   Your **mass** is the same on any planet.

5. That is why you *weigh* more on Jupiter than you do on Earth. Your mass is the same in both places. But because of the stronger force of gravity, you weigh more on Jupiter.

6. Note that mass is the same on Mercury, Jupiter, Mars, or any other planet. Your *weight* on these planets will be different.

7.7

Problem 5:

Which free-falling object has the greater force from gravity imposed on it, a 15-kg watermelon or a 20-kg rock?

A) The watermelon

B) The rock

C) Both items are subject to the exact same force, 9.8 N.

D) Both items are subject to the exact same force, 19.6 N.

STRATEGY

Use the equation, $F = mg$.

THINK

- $F_{melon} = m_{melon} \cdot g$ $F_{rock} = m_{rock} \cdot g$

    $= 15 \,\cancel{kg} \cdot 9.8$ $N/\cancel{kg} = 20 \,\cancel{kg} \cdot 9.8 \,N/\cancel{kg}$

    $= 147 \,N$ $= 196 \,N$

- The force on the rock is greater because it has greater mass.

- Note that although the *acceleration* of both objects is the same (ignoring air resistance), the force on the objects is not the same. Force is proportional to mass—the greater the mass an object has, the greater force that gravity applies to it.

7.7

Problem 6:

A dog weighs 40 lb on Earth. How much will the dog weigh on Jupiter?

A) 15.2 lb   B) 40 lb   C) 42.6 lb   D) 52 lb

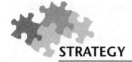

STRATEGY

Find the weight by multiplying by the gravitational strength for Jupiter.

THINK

- The force of gravity on Jupiter is 2.6 times as strong as the force of gravity on Earth. Therefore:

- $W_{Jupiter} = W_{Earth} \cdot 2.6$

  $= 40 \cdot 2.6$

  $= 52 \text{ lb}$

- The dog would weigh 52 lb on Jupiter, making (D) the correct response.

F. Momentum

1. **Momentum** is a vector quantity (includes direction) that measures a combination of an object's size and velocity:

   $p = m \cdot v$

   where p stands for momentum and m and v stand for mass and velocity.

2. Momentum is "mass in motion" and is directly proportional to mass.

3. When two objects, such as football players, collide, the object with the greater momentum will push the other object back.

4. Thus, a small football player moving very fast can knock over a large, slow football player because the small player has greater momentum.

5. Force applied over time is known as **impulse**. The impulse equation comes from the force equation.

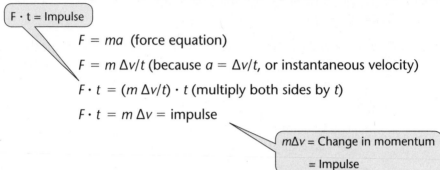

$F \cdot t = \text{Impulse}$

$F = ma$ (force equation)

$F = m \, \Delta v/t$ (because $a = \Delta v/t$, or instantaneous velocity)

$F \cdot t = (m \, \Delta v/t) \cdot t$ (multiply both sides by t)

$F \cdot t = m \, \Delta v = \text{impulse}$

$m\Delta v = \text{Change in momentum}$
$= \text{Impulse}$

6. So impulse equals $F \cdot t$, or the change in momentum. Whereas impulse is typically measured in *N-s*, change in momentum has units of *kg-m/s*.

7. Note that increasing t in an impulse reduces the amount of force applied to an object. This is what padding does for a football helmet. The padding slows down the impact over a longer period of time, thereby reducing the force to the head.

7.7

Problem 7:

To give her stroke the greatest force, a tennis player can hit the ball with an impulse of 1 *N-s*. Which stroke will give the most force, a short, quick stroke of 0.1 s or a longer stroke of 0.2 s?

A) The shorter stroke produces a greater force of 10 *N*.

B) The longer stroke produces a greater force of 10 *N*.

C) The shorter stroke produces a greater force of 5 *N*.

D) The longer stroke produces a greater force of 5 *N*.

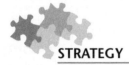

STRATEGY

Refer to the definition of impulse $= F \cdot t$.

THINK

- Impulse $= F \cdot t$, so for an impulse of 1 *N-s*, for the short stroke:

$$1 \text{ } N\text{-}s = F \cdot (0.1 \text{ } s)$$
$$F = 10 \text{ } N$$

- For the long stroke:

$$1 \text{ } N\text{-}s = F \cdot (0.2 \text{ } s)$$
$$F = 5 \text{ } N$$

- The short stroke clearly has more force, so answer choice (A) is the correct response.

G. Conservation of Momentum

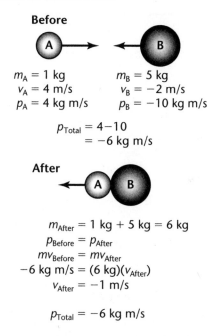

Before

$m_A = 1$ kg $m_B = 5$ kg
$v_A = 4$ m/s $v_B = -2$ m/s
$p_A = 4$ kg m/s $p_B = -10$ kg m/s

$$p_{Total} = 4-10$$
$$= -6 \text{ kg m/s}$$

After

$$m_{After} = 1 \text{ kg} + 5 \text{ kg} = 6 \text{ kg}$$
$$p_{Before} = p_{After}$$
$$mv_{Before} = mv_{After}$$
$$-6 \text{ kg m/s} = (6 \text{ kg})(v_{After})$$
$$v_{After} = -1 \text{ m/s}$$

$$p_{Total} = -6 \text{ kg m/s}$$

1. Newton's third law (above) states that for every action there is an equal and opposite reaction.

2. That means in a collision between ball A and ball B:

   a. The force on each ball is equal: $F_A = F_B$

   b. The time of collision is equal: $t_A = t_B$

c. The total momentum of the balls is conserved both before and after the collision. No momentum is lost.

d. After the collision, both balls move to the left at a speed of -1 m/s.

7.2

Problem 8:

Football linebacker A has mass of 100 kg and moves at velocity of -2.8 m/s (west). Running back B has mass of 60 kg and moves at velocity of 10 m/s (east). After the two collide, in which direction and at what speed will they move as a pair?

A) 2 m/s west   B) 2 m/s east   C) 5 m/s east   D) 3 m/s west

STRATEGY

The total momentum of both players must be the same both before and after the collision.

THINK

- Find the momentum of each player before the collision.

$$p_A = m_A \cdot v_A \qquad\qquad p_B = m_B \cdot v_B$$
$$= (100)(-2.8) \qquad\qquad = (60)(10)$$
$$= -280 \text{ kg} - \text{m/s} \qquad = 600 \text{ kg} - \text{m/s}$$
$$p_{Before} = -280 + 600$$
$$= 320 \text{ kg} - \text{m/s}$$

- Now, p_{Before} must be equal to p_{After} so:

$$mv_{Before} = mv_{After}$$
$$320 \text{ kg-m/s} = (100 + 60)(v_{After})$$
$$v_{After} = 2 \text{ m/s}$$

- So both players move east at a speed of 2 m/s, making (B) the correct response.

| 7.8 | **ENERGY AND WORK** |

A. Work

1. **Work** requires a force that must cause a displacement.

2. A person pushes against a refrigerator, but the refrigerator does not budge. Is work done? No, because although force was applied, there was no displacement of the refrigerator.

3. A weightlifter holds a 50-kg dumbbell off the ground. Is work done? Yes, because the weightlifter applies force and the bar moves, a displacement occurs.

> Note: Work and energy have the same units, joules. (See section 7.8 B.)

4. Work is measured in **joules** (J).

   1 joule = 1 newton-meter = 1 $N \cdot$ 1 m = $1kg - m^2/s^2$

7.8

Problem 1:

A weightlifter holds a 50-kg bar steadily in place over her head. Is work done while she is holding the bar in place?

A) Yes, she is doing work by keeping the bar from falling.

B) Yes, she is doing work because she is applying force to the bar.

C) No, she is not doing work because she not applying force to the bar.

D) No, she is not doing work because the bar is not displaced.

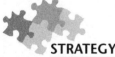

STRATEGY

Apply the concept of work to the situation.

THINK

- To do work, the weightlifter must apply force, and the force must cause a displacement.

- The weightlifter is clearly applying force. However, the bar is not changing position (displacement). Therefore, no work is being done, making (D) the correct response.

B. Potential Energy

1. **Energy** is the ability to do work.

2. Energy comes in many forms, including potential (stored) energy, kinetic (motion) energy, mechanical energy, electrical energy, electromagnetic energy, and many others.

3. Energy is measured in the same units as work, Joules, where $1 J = 1$ newton-meter.

4. **Potential energy** (PE) is the energy that is stored as a result of an object's position.

5. An example of positional energy is the energy stored in a stretched rubber band.

6. The force of gravity gives objects PE as a result of their position or height off the ground.
   $$PE = Mass \cdot g \cdot Height \quad (g = 9.8 \ N \ / \ kg)$$
   $$= m \cdot g \cdot h$$

7.8

Problem 2:

A 50-kg woman on the third floor of a building takes the elevator the second floor and gets out. By how much does her potential energy change if each floor is 10 m in height?

A) 24,500 J   C) −4900 J

B) −9800 J   D) 14,700 J

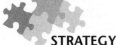

STRATEGY

Use the formula for PE to find the amount of PE the woman has both initially and after she has gotten off the elevator.

THINK

- The woman's PE is calculated using $PE = m \cdot g \cdot h$ for any position.
- Her change in PE is calculated by subtracting $PE_{final} - PE_{initial}$.
- $$PE_{initial} = m \cdot g \cdot h$$
  $$= (50)(9.8)(30 \text{ m})$$
  $$= 14{,}700 \text{ J}$$
  $$PE_{final} = (50)(9.8)(20 \text{ m})$$
  $$= 9800 \text{ J}$$
  $$\Delta PE = 9800 - 14{,}700$$
  $$= -4900 \text{ J}$$

- The PE of the woman decreases because she goes from a higher floor to a lower floor. Therefore, answer choice (C) is correct.

C. Kinetic Energy

1. **Kinetic energy** (KE) is the energy that an object has when it is in motion. KE is given by:

   $KE = 1/2\ mv^2$

   where m is the mass of the object and v is its speed.

2. KE, similar to all forms of energy, is measured in joules, the same units that are used for work. $1\ J = 1\ N{-}m = 1\ kg{-}m^2/s^2$

3. KE is a scalar quantity. Unlike velocity, momentum, or acceleration, KE has no direction.

4. KE is proportional to the square of its speed. Doubling the speed of an object increases its KE by a factor of 2^2 or 4.

5. The kind of KE that can do work—apply forces that cause displacements—is **mechanical energy**.

6. The figure of a ball dropping on ice shows how PE, KE, and work are different.

   a. PE involves raising the heavy ball to height *h* over the ice.

   b. PE is converted to KE when the ball drops and is moving.

   c. The KE is converted to mechanical energy that does work by displacing the ice.

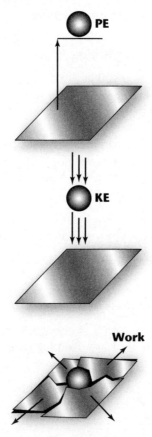

7. Similar to momentum, energy is always conserved. Energy cannot be created or destroyed. It can only be converted from one form of energy to another.

8. The diagram shows how energy can be converted from one form to others.

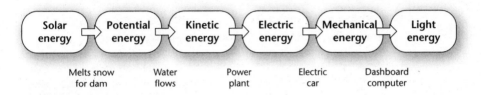

| Solar energy | Potential energy | Kinetic energy | Electric energy | Mechanical energy | Light energy |

Melts snow for dam · Water flows · Power plant · Electric car · Dashboard computer

7.8

Problem 3:

Warm weather increases the speed of air particles inside of a rubber tire by 150%. By how much does the kinetic energy of the particles increase?

A) 150%   B) 225%   C) 22.5%   D) 400%

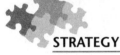

STRATEGY

Refer to the relationship between the speed of the object and its KE.

THINK

- $KE_{initial} = 1/2\ m(v_{initial})^2$
- Assume $v_{initial} = 1$. Then $v_{final} = 150\%$ of 1 or: $1.5 \times 1 = 1.5$.
- $KE_{final}/KE_{initial} = 1/2\ m(1.5)^2 / 1/2\ m(1)^2$
  = 2.25
- $2.25 \times 100 = 225\%$
- This means that (B) is the correct answer choice.

7.9   ELECTRICITY

A. Charge and Current

1. The attraction between positive protons and negative electrons keeps neutral atoms together. However, these charges can be separated.

2. Rubbing a balloon with fur strips electrons creates **static electricity**, giving the balloon a negative charge.

3. In a battery (electrochemical cell), a reaction takes place that causes electrons to flow in **electric current** from the negative terminal to the positive terminal.

> A battery is actually a series of electrochemical cells.

> A battery turns chemical energy into electric energy.

4. Energy in a battery is measured in **volts**. Electrons in a 12-volt battery are more strongly attracted to the positive terminal and can do more work than electrons in a 6-volt battery.

5. Each bulb or device in a **circuit** has **resistance** to electron flow and consumes energy when current flows through it.

6. The relationship between voltage (V, volts), current (I, amperes), and **resistance** (R, ohms) is given in Ohm's law. For this circuit:

   $V = IR$ (Ohm's law)

   $12\ V = (3\ ohms) \cdot (4\ amps)$

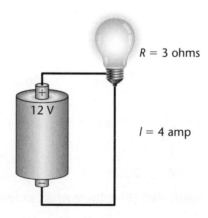

$R = 3$ ohms

12 V

$I = 4$ amp

7.9

Problem 1:

What current flows through this circuit?

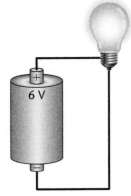

$R = 2.5$ ohms

6 V

$I = ?$

A) 8.5 amps

B) 2.4 amps

C) 3.5 volts

D) 15 ohms

STRATEGY

Use Ohm's law.

THINK

- $V = IR$

  $6 V = I (2.5)$

  $I = 2.4$ amps

- The simple *relationship* in Ohm's law allows you to compute any resistance, voltage, or current. In this case, (B) is the correct response.

B. Series and Parallel Circuits

1. A **series** of cells forms a **battery**. The voltage of this series equals the sum of cells:

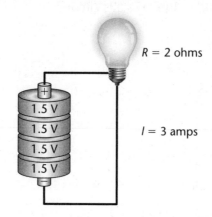

R = 2 ohms

1.5 V
1.5 V
1.5 V
1.5 V

I = 3 amps

$V = 1.5 + 1.5 + 1.5 + 1.5 = 6\ V$

2. Devices in a circuit can also be set up in series.

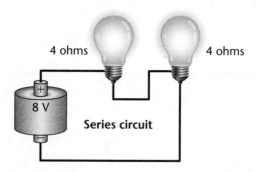

4 ohms   4 ohms

8 V

Series circuit

3. This series circuit has a total resistance of:

$R = 4 + 4 = 8$ ohms

4. So the current in the above series circuit is:

$V = IR$ so:

$I = R/V$

$= 8$ ohms $/ 8\ V = 1.0$ amp

5. In a **parallel** circuit, both pathways obtain the full 8 V voltage of the circuit. With both paths open, resistance drops and current increases.

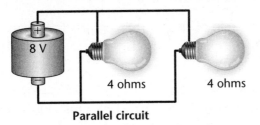

Parallel circuit

6. The table below compares the series and parallel circuits above.

	Series	Parallel
Voltage	8 V	8 V (each path)
Adding bulbs (resistors)	Current decreases	Current increases
Adding bulbs (resistors)	Overall resistance increases	Overall resistance decreases
Current	All bulbs have same current	Paths share current; different paths have different current
One bulb goes out	Whole series goes dark	Path goes dark, but other path stays lit

7.9

Problem 2:

A bulb on the hospital Christmas tree blows, and the entire tree goes dark. Joy then replaces the bulb, and the lights go on. What can be said about the current flowing through each bulb in the Christmas tree circuit?

A) The current is different for each path in the circuit.

B) The current is the same for each bulb in the circuit.

C) The first bulb in the circuit has the greatest amount of current.

D) The last bulb in the circuit has the greatest amount of current.

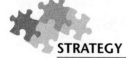

STRATEGY

Determine the kind of circuit. Then use its characteristics to draw a conclusion.

THINK

- The entire tree went dark when a bulb blew out. This means that the tree has a series circuit.
- For a series circuit, each resistor (bulb) has the same amount of current flowing through it. Therefore, answer choice (B) is correct.

Glossary

abiotic: The nonbiological factors in an ecosystem, such as air, water, soil, and rock

absolute value: A bracket function that turns any value within its brackets positive; for example, $|-27| = 27$

acid: A sour, corrosive chemical that ionizes in water to form H^+ ions and has a pH of below 7.0

adaptation: In evolution, a change in form brought about by a mutation that results in an advantage for an organism; for example, a white coat is a useful adaptation for a polar bear

adjective: A word that modifies a noun or pronoun; for example, a *red* coat, a *small* dog

adverb: A word that modifies a verb, adjective, or another adverb; for example, Al *quickly* smiled. Jane walks *slowly*.

allele: A form of a gene that codes for a specific trait; for example, Mendel's peas had a dominant *tall* allele and a recessive *short* allele

amino acid: One of 20 small nitrogen-containing organic acid that serves as a building block for all proteins

antecedent: In grammar, the noun that the pronoun refers to; for example, *him* may refer to the antecedent *Charles*

antibody: A blood protein that is made by B cells to bind to foreign antigens that enter the body so they can be eliminated

antigen: A toxin or foreign substance that produces an immune response in the body; for example, the immune response might be the production of antibodies

apostrophe: A punctuation mark that shows ownership and identifies missing letters in contractions

artery: A blood vessel that carries blood *away* from the heart; typically, arteries carry red blood, but the pulmonary artery that goes from the heart to the lungs carries blue blood

atom: The fundamental unit of matter that makes up the 118 different elements, or forms of matter that exist, that consists of a central nucleus containing protons, neutrons, and outer electrons

atomic mass: The mass of a single atom in amu units

atomic number: The number that identifies a particular species of an atom on the periodic table and tells how many protons and electrons that the primary isotope of that atom has; for example, with atomic number 6, carbon has 6 protons and 6 electrons

atomic radius: The distance from an atom's nucleus to its outermost electron

atrium: One of the top chambers of the heart that receives blood from the body

author's purpose: The aim of the author in writing the text; typically to explain, persuade, entertain, or express feelings

axon: The long, thin, conductive part of the neuron that brings electrical information away from the neuron cell body

B cells: A type of white blood cell that produces antibodies

base: A chemical that produces OH^{-1} ions in solution, has a pH of greater than 7.0, and reacts with acids

bases: One of the four "alphabet letters" that make up the genetic code for DNA: A (adenine), T (thymine), C (cytosine), and G (guanine)

battery: An electrochemical cell; technically, a battery is more than one cell connected in series

bias: A prejudice that is typically based on a faulty opinion

biome: One of Earth's major biological regions; for example, grassland, tundra, or desert

biotic: A factor in an ecosystem that is biological in origin such as plants, animals, or fungus

capillary: A very tiny blood vessel that can either be an artery or a vein

cause and effect: A text structure in which the cause of an event directly precedes the outcome of the event, or its effect

cell: The basic biological unit of all living things

cellular respiration: The process of cells burning oxygen to obtain energy and give off carbon dioxide as a waste product

central nervous system: The part of the nervous system that includes the brain and spinal cord

chemical change: A change in the composition of atoms or molecules

as a result of a chemical reaction; for example, when H_2O is broken into H_2 and O_2, the composition of atoms has changed

chromosomes: Structures in the cell nucleus that are made of DNA and contain the genetic code for an organism; humans have 23 pairs of chromosomes

circuit: An electrical system in which current flows in a circular path

circulatory system: The body system that includes the heart and blood vessels

clause: A group of words that include a noun and a verb

colon: The punctuation mark (:) that typically introduces a list

comma splice: A construction that incorrectly combines two sentences into a single sentence that are separated by a comma; comma splices should not be found in a well-written text

command: A sentence that gives an order or makes a request

comma: The punctuation mark (,) that signals a pause in the text

community: All of the different species of organisms that exist in a particular area of ecosystem

compare and contrast: A text structure in which an item is introduced in one section and then compared with another item in the following section

compound: A pure substance such as methane (CH_4) or water (H_2O), that is made of a single type of molecule

concentration: The amount of solute that is dissolved in a solution; a solution with a high concentration has a large amount of solute dissolved

conclusion: A judgment or decision that a reader draws from reading a text

consumers: Biological organisms that cannot make their own food such as animals or fungi

context: The text that surrounds a particular item or passage in a text and gives it background meaning

context clues: Hints about the meaning of a text that are derived from assessing its surrounding words, or context

coordinating conjunction: The words that include *and, so, but, for, or, nor,* and *yet* that are used to connect two independent clauses

covalent bonds: Chemical bonds in which electrons are shared equally

dash: The punctuation mark (—) that is used to introduce a surprise or to set off important information

declarative: A sentence that states a fact or makes a statement

dendrites: The parts of a neuron that receives input from other neurons

denominator: The bottom part of a fraction

dependent clause: A clause that cannot stand on its own; for example, the italicized words in the following sentence comprise a dependent clause: *When the rain stopped,* Jo went home

diabetes: A disease in which person does not secrete a sufficient amount of insulin into the bloodstream, so his or her body cells become "starved" because they cannot take in glucose

diffusion: The process in which material flows from a more concentrated area (e.g., in a solution) to an area that is less concentrated

digestive system: The body system that breaks down food and delivers it to the bloodstream

displacement: A change of position, typically the result of movement

divisor: In division, the number that divides into a second number; for $24 \div 3$ the number 3 is the divisor

DNA: The genetic molecule that makes up chromosomes in the cells and forms the genetic code; DNA codes for the proteins that help carry out all important life processes

dominant: In genetics, an allele with a trait that prevails when it is present and the other allele is recessive; for example, a *tall* allele can be dominant over a *short* allele

double replacement: A chemical reaction in which two components switch places as in $AB + CD * AD + CB$

drawing a conclusion: Using evidence and reasoning in a text to make a deduction

ecosystem: An environment that includes both biotic (e.g., plants, animals) and abiotic (e.g., air, soil, water) factors

electric current: The movement of electrons

electronegativity: The tendency of an atom to attract electrons

electrons: Negatively charged fundamental particles that exist outside of the nucleus of every atom

element: A substance, such as carbon, nickel, or chlorine, that is made of a single type of atom

embryo: A growing organism that is incomplete and unborn

endocrine: Pertaining to hormones

endothermic: A reaction that takes in energy

energy: The ability to do work

entertain: One of the four purposes for which an author writes a text, which include to explain, persuade, entertain, or express feelings

enzyme: A protein that facilitates a chemical reaction

estimate: In math, to find an approximate answer

evolution: The process by which biological organisms change in form over time because of adaptations that produce different levels of survivability within an environment

exclamatory: A sentence that expresses excitement or surprise.

excretory system: The body system that gets rid of cellular waste that is expelled from the body after being processed in the kidneys

exothermic: A reaction that gives off energy

experiment: A scientific procedure that is undertaken to test a hypothesis or answer a question

explain: One of the four purposes for which an author writes a text, which include to explain, persuade, entertain, or express feelings

expository: A sentence or passage that explains

express feelings: One of the four purposes for which an author writes a text, which include to explain, persuade, entertain, or express feelings

$F = ma$: An expression of Newton's second law in which force (F) is equal to mass (m) times acceleration (a)

factor: A number that when multiplied by another factor equals a third number; 3 and 5 are both factors of 15 because $3 \times 5 = 15$

fact: A description that can be supported by logic and evidence

first person: A sentence told from the "I" or "me" point of view

FOIL method: A method of factoring polynomials in which the first factors are followed by the outside factors, the inside factors, and the last factors

food web: A diagram that shows energy relationships among different organisms in an ecosystem

force: A measure of mass times acceleration

fractions: numbers that are expressed in rational form with a numerator over a denominator

gas: The state of matter in which atoms or molecules move freely as a fluid and fill up any space that they inhabit

GCF (greatest common factor): The factor of two numbers that is greatest in value; the GCF of 8 and 12 is 4 because 4 is the greatest number that divides equally into both 8 and 12

gene: A section of a chromosome; typically a gene codes for a particular protein

genotype: The genetic make-up of an organism with regard to its alleles; the genotype of an organism with dominant and recessive "T" and "S" genes might be TtSs; another individual might have genotype ttSs

glomerulus: A functional unit of the kidney that controls excretion

homeostasis: The tendency of an organism to find a safe, stable state for all body functions within its internal environment

hormones: Chemicals such as testosterone that are secreted by glands, distributed through the blood, and facilitate activity and change in other parts of the body

hypertonic: An area in which matter is concentrated and tends to diffuse to a less concentrated area

hyphen: The small, dash-like punctuation mark ($-$) that is used to join words that themselves are used to modify, such as the mark that joins "dash-like" here

hypothesis: A proposed explanation for a scientific phenomenon that can be tested in an experiment

hypotonic: An area in which a substance is less concentrated; the substance tends to diffuse into a hypotonic area from an area of higher concentration

improper fraction: A fraction in which the numerator is greater than the denominator

impulse: Force applied over a period of time

Independent clause: A clause that can stand on its own as a complete sentence; in the following sentence, both clauses are independent: Ralph was hungry, so he bought a sandwich.

inertia: An expression of Newton's first law; the tendency of an object to stay in motion at a constant velocity unless it is acted on by an outside force

inference: An educated guess that a reader makes about a text based on evidence within the text, logic, and personal experience

ingredients label: A label on a food product that reveals the food's nutritional composition

insulin: A hormone secreted by the pancreas that makes it possible for blood glucose to enter body cells

integers: Whole numbers that are both positive and negative and include zero

interrogative: A sentence that asks a question

ionic bond: A chemical bond between ions such as Na^+ and Cl^- in which the negative ion completely "captures" the electron from the positive ion

ionization energy: The energy required to remove an atom's outermost electron

ions: Atoms that take on extra electrons or give up an electron; ions typically exist in solution such as NaCl breaking up into as Na^+ and Cl^- ions in water

isotopes: Atom species that contain a particular number of neutrons and therefore have particular atomic mass; isotopes of carbon include C^{14} and C^{12}; Rare C^{14} is typically called the "isotope" even though both forms properly should be called isotopes

killer T cells: Cells in the immune system that kill off foreign cells in the body that are identified by helper cells

kinetic energy: The energy of an object in motion

kingdom: One of the six divisions of biological organisms that include bacteria, Archaeobacteria, plants, animals, fungi, and protists

large intestine: The lower portion of the body's digestive system that concentrates waste and delivers it so it can be expelled from the body

LCD (lowest common denominator): Denominator of lowest value that can express two fractions; for example, 24 is the LCD for 5/12 and 3/8 because 24 is the lowest number that can be used as a denominator for both fractions: 5/12 = 10/**24**; 3/8 = 9/**24**

LCM (least common multiple): Lowest valued multiple of two numbers; for example, 24 is the LCM for 12 and 8 because 24 is the lowest number that is a multiple of 12 and 8

like terms: In algebra, two terms that have the same variable to the same power that can be combined using addition or subtraction

liquid: The state of matter in which particles are attracted but still can move somewhat freely

litmus paper: Paper used to determine the pH (acidity) of a chemical

lungs: Organs in the human body used for breathing, taking in oxygen and expelling carbon dioxide

main idea: The primary point in a text; the reason that a text is written

mechanical energy: Energy that is used to do work on real items such as a piston in an engine

median: The middle value a data set; in a set of 7 values, the median would be the fourth value, whatever that is

meiosis: Process in which gametes (egg and sperm cells) are formed that have only a single set ($1n$) of chromosomes rather than the normal double ($2n$) set of chromosomes that all other body cells have

mental math: Calculation process that is carried out mentally without paper

pencil or a mechanical or electronic calculating device

mitosis: Process in which cells divide to grow

mixture: A blend of particles

mode: The most common value in a data set

molarity: The number of moles of a chemical per liter of solution; a solution of $2M$ contains 2 moles of the chemical for every liter of solution

mole: 6.02×10^{23} particles of a substance; for example, a mole of carbon has 6.02×10^{23} atoms and a mass of exactly 12 grams; a mole of oxygen has 6.02×10^{23} molecules and a mass of exactly 32 grams

molecule: A pure substance that consists of atoms that are bonded to one another; for example, water consists of molecules of H_2O; nitrogen consists of molecules of N_2

momentum: An object's mass multiplied by its velocity

musculoskeletal system: Body system that includes the muscles and bones and is used for movement

mutation: A mistake in the copying of DNA that usually results in faulty proteins that are lethal but can sometimes result in beneficial adaptations

narrative: A text that has a story form

natural selection: In evolution, the process by organisms that are fittest for their environment are selected and survive more readily than other organisms; natural selection singled out polar bears in Arctic to survive, presumably because their white coat gave them an advantage over darker bears

negative number: Any number that is less than zero

nephrons: Units of the excretory system within the kidney

neurons: Nerve cells

neurotransmitters: Chemicals released in a synapse between neurons that chemically transmit an electrical nerve signal from one neuron to the next neuron

neutrons: Particles in the nucleus of an atom that have a mass of 1 amu but no charge

Newton's first law: Law that states that all objects have inertia, which causes them to stay in motion at the same speed (which can be moving or at rest) in the same direction unless they are acted on by an unbalanced force

Newton's second law: The law that states that force (F) is equal to mass (m) times acceleration (a)

noun: A word that names a person, place, thing, or idea

nucleus: 1. Center part of an atom that contains protons and neutrons; 2. In a cell the part of the cell that contains chromosomes and DNA

number facts: Basic addition, subtraction, multiplication, and division facts

number line: Line that includes all numbers

numerator: Top part of a fraction

operation: Addition, subtraction, multiplication, or division

opinion: A statement that reflects a person's personal judgment, which may or may not be supported by evidence or facts

opinion: Personal view that may or may not be supported by facts

order of operations: Protocol in algebra in which operations are carried out

organelles: Discrete structures in cells such as mitochondria, the nucleus, Golgi bodies, and chloroplasts

organic: Chemical that contains carbon

organ: Highly organized body part such as the heart, brain, or liver that performs a specific function or group of functions

ovaries: Female organs that produce eggs

parallel: Two lines that never meet

passive voice: A sentence or text in which the initiator of the action is not clearly identified; for example, *Mistakes were made*

past participle: The verb form used with helping verbs (*have*) such as *eaten, brought,* and *heard*

period: Punctuation mark (.) that ends a declarative sentence

periodic table: In chemistry, the table that organizes all 118 known elements into groups with similar properties

peristalsis: Muscular process by which food in the digestive system is moved through the system

personal pronoun: Pronoun that stands for a person, such as *I, you,* or *she*

persuasive: The type of writing that attempts to convince the reader to take a position or do something

pH: Log scale that measures the acidity of a substance; whereas low pH indicates high acidity, high pH indicates low acidity (highly basic)

phenotype: The body form of an organism as opposed to its genotype; when T is dominant for "tall," an individual with "tall" phenotype may have genotype TT or Tt

photosynthesis: The process by which plants and other organisms use sunlight and carbon dioxide to produce sugars

phrase: A group of words that does not include both a subject or predicate

physical changes: Changes that do not involve a change in chemical composition; ice melting is a physical change because H_2O does not change chemical composition during melting

place value: Value of a place in the number system; the 4 in the number 846 shows that there are 4 tens or 40 in the *tens* column

population: Number of an individual species in a community such as the population of bullfrogs in a pond

possessive pronouns: Pronoun that shows possession such as *hers, yours,* or *mine*

potential energy: The energy that is stored as a result of an object's position

predicate: The "verb" part of a sentence that expresses action or being

prediction: A guess made by the reader about future events or actions

preposition: Small words such as *for, in, at, from,* that always take an object and define relationships between other words and phrases in a sentence

present participle: The verb form used with helping verbs (*be*) that show

ongoing action as *eating, bringing,* or *hearing*

problem-solution: Text structure in which problems are posed and are followed by solutions

producers: In a biological community, the photosynthesizing food makers such as plants and algae

product: The "answer" in multiplication

pronoun: A word such as *he, she, it,* or *me* that takes the place of a noun

proper noun: A noun that names a person, place, or thing that is always capitalized, such as Arizona and Donald Draper

proportion: Special algebraic equation in which two fractions are set equal to one another

protein: Body chemicals that perform an enormous number of disparate functions, some of which are structural; many proteins function as enzymes that facilitate otherwise "impossible" chemical reactions that allow life processes such as metabolism to be carried out

protons: Positive particles in the nucleus of an atom that have atomic mass of 1 amu

quotation marks: Punctuation that identifies the exact words of a speaker

quotient: The "answer" in division; in $40 \div 5 = 8$, the 8 is the quotient

ratio: Relationship between two numbers as in a fraction; 4/5 is a ratio that can be written as 4 to 5, 4:5 or 4 out of 5

recessive: In genetics, a trait that is expressed only when both alleles are identical and recessive; if only one allele is recessive then the trait is not expressed; for example, if *T* is dominant for tall and *t* is recessive for short, a *Tt* individual is tall, and only a *tt* individual is short

reciprocal: A fraction that is turned "upside down" in which the numerator and denominator switch places

reliability: A scientific procedure or experiment that is repeatable over time

resistance: In an electric circuit, how difficult it is for current to flow; resistance is a measure of how much energy is lost as a current flows through a part of the circuit; for example, a toaster, uses resistance to convert electric current into heat energy

respiration: The process by which oxygen is used to break down food (e.g., sugar) and produce energy in the form of adenosine triphosphate (ATP) molecules

RNA: In cells, nucleic acids that carry out protein synthesis, expressing the code inscribed in DNA

rounding: In math, approximating a number; for example, 48 rounded to the nearest ten is 50

run-on: A construction that contains two independent clauses that should be broken up into two separate sentences

second person: A sentence that addresses *you*

semicolon: A punctuation mark (;) that is used to separate independent clauses that are not connected by a conjunction (and other purposes)

sentence: A group of words that includes a subject and predicate and expresses a complete thought

sentence fragment: A sentence-like construction that is incomplete in some way and therefore does not qualify as a sentence

sequence: A text structure that can take the form of a list, numbered steps, a bulleted list, or a series in outline form

series: A group of items that are connected in some consecutive way

sign: The designation of positive ($+$) or negative ($-$) on an integer

simple sentence: A sentence that contains only a subject and a verb and has no clauses or phrases

simplest terms: A fraction that exists in smallest whole number terms with both numerator and denominator having their smallest possible value

single replacement: A chemical reaction in which one component switches for another as in AB + C * AC + B

slope: The ratio of rise to run in a graph calculated by the ratio of Δy to Δx; a graph with a high positive slope appears to rise sharply from left to right

small intestine: Part of the body's digestive system in which food is broken down into its smallest form and absorbed into the bloodstream

solid: State of matter in which particles are "frozen" into place and cannot move freely past one another

solubility: How readily a substance dissolves

solute: The substance that dissolves in a solution; in salt water, salt is the solute

solution: A homogeneous mixture in which solute particles such as salt completely disappear within the solvent (e.g., water)

solvent: The medium in a solution; in salt water, water is the solvent

static electricity: Form of electricity in which charge builds up and can flow across a nonconductor such as air

stereotype: An oversimplified and often incorrect view of a member of a group; for example, "hardworking" is a common stereotype for Asians

subject: The item that a phrase or a sentence is about

sum: The "answer" in math when quantities are added

summarizing: A brief, condensed accounting of a longer text

supporting detail: A fact or item within a text that supports a main idea

synthesis: Process in which two (or more) items are combined to form a single item

testosterone: Male sex hormone

text structure: Text that has a particular format such as sequence, problem–solution, or cause and effect

theme: A text's highest and most general subject; themes are typically "big" ideas such as love, beauty, or the meaning of friendship

third person: Text written from the "he," "she," and "they" point of view

tissues: Cells that are joined together for a single function, such as muscle tissue

topic: The subject of a text

topic sentence: Sentence that typically contains the main idea of a paragraph

unlike terms: Algebraic terms that cannot be combined using addition or subtraction because they do not share the same variable to the same power

uterus: Part of the female reproductive system in which fertilized eggs implant and grow into embryos, eventually developing into fetuses

vaccine: A weakened form of an antigen that is deliberately introduced into the body to activate the production of antibodies to prevent disease

valence electrons: The outermost electrons in an atom that are typically lost or gained when the atom forms an ion

validity: A scientific procedure or experiment has validity if it is able to measure the quantity or quality that is intended to be measured

variable: In algebra, a letter quantity that can stand for any number or quantity

veins: Blood vessels that carry blood to the heart; typically, veins carry blue blood, but the pulmonary vein that goes from the lungs to the heart carries red blood

velocity: A measure of the speed and direction of a moving object

ventricles: The lower chambers of the heart

verb: An action word or a word of being; for example, *run, eat,* or *be*

volts: A measurement of energy in a battery or electrical system; a system with greater voltage has greater electrical "pressure" for electrons to move and current to flow

work: What occurs when a force produces a displacement; work is measured in units of energy

zygote: A fertilized egg that has not yet begun to divide

Notes

Notes

Notes

Notes

Notes

Notes

Notes

Notes